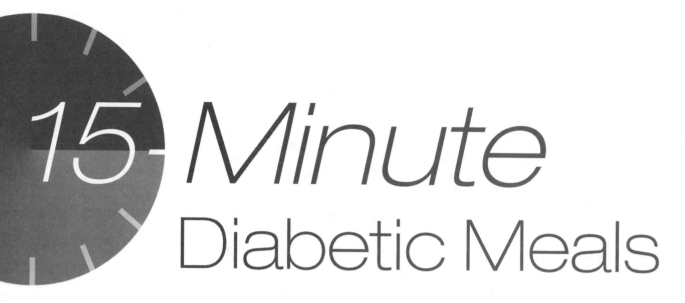

15 *Minute*
Diabetic Meals

By Nancy S. Hughes

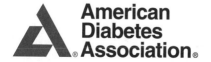

American Diabetes Association

Director, Book Publishing, Robert Anthony; *Managing Editor,* Abe Ogden; *Acquisitions Editor,* Victor Van Beuren; *Production Manager,* Melissa Sprott; *Composition,* ADA; *Cover Design,* Vis-á-Vis Creative Concepts; *Photography,* Burwell and Burwell Photography.

Printed in Canada
1 3 5 7 9 10 8 6 4 2

The suggestions and information contained in this publication are generally consistent with the Clinical Practice Recommendations and other policies of the American Diabetes Association, but they do not represent the policy or position of the Association or any of its boards or committees. Reasonable steps have been taken to ensure the accuracy of the information presented. However, the American Diabetes Association cannot ensure the safety or efficacy of any product or service described in this publication. Individuals are advised to consult a physician or other appropriate health care professional before undertaking any diet or exercise program or taking any medication referred to in this publication. Professionals must use and apply their own professional judgment, experience, and training and should not rely solely on the information contained in this publication before prescribing any diet, exercise, or medication. The American Diabetes Association—its officers, directors, employees, volunteers, and members—assumes no responsibility or liability for personal or other injury, loss, or damage that may result from the suggestions or information in this publication.

⊚ The paper in this publication meets the requirements of the ANSI Standard Z39.48-1992 (permanence of paper).

ADA titles may be purchased for business or promotional use or for special sales. To purchase more than 50 copies of this book at a discount, or for custom editions of this book with your logo, contact the American Diabetes Association at the address below, at booksales@diabetes.org, or by calling 703-299-2046.

American Diabetes Association
1701 North Beauregard Street
Alexandria, Virginia 22311

DOI: 10.2337/9781580403207

Library of Congress Cataloging-in-Publication Data
Hughes, Nancy S.
  15-minute diabetic meals / Nancy S. Hughes.
     p. cm.
  Includes bibliographical references and index.
  ISBN 978-1-58040-320-7 (alk. paper)
1. Diabetes--Diet therapy--Recipes. 2. Quick and easy cookery. I. Title. II. Title: Fifteen-minute diabetic meals.
  RC662.H835 2010
  641.5'6314--dc22
                              2010001833

This book is dedicated to my husband, Greg:
You're funny when I need a laugh,
you're brilliant when I need a mind,
you're definitely fun to be around during
the chaos and the deadlines in my business!

Thanks, I need every bit of that!

And

To my children and their growing families:
Will, Kelly, Molly Catherine, Anna Flynn, Annie, and Taft.
This family is exploding—and I love it, absolutely love it!
Thanks for tasting the food when you're around, listening
about the food when you're not—and always being hungry
for what's next!

TABLE OF CONTENTS

PREFACE

Does this sound familiar? It's 6:30 a.m. and you're scrambling, so you grab a piece of toast on your way out the door. Four and a half hours later you find yourself in that fast food line, thinking you'll do better at dinner. It's 5:20 p.m. and you don't have a clue what to fix for dinner, so you order take-out and promise yourself you'll do better tomorrow. But invariably it starts all over the next day, and the next day, and the next. As your wallet shrinks, so does your nutrition.

How can you get out of this vicious cycle? By taking charge—and having fun while you're at it!

The secret to healthier eating is having nutritious ingredients on hand for super-fast meals without a lot of effort or expense, while getting rid of the junk food lurking behind those kitchen doors. Pitch it out, give it away, or simply just don't buy more junk. Don't make it a big deal; just do it. Then restock your shelves with items you actually like and will want to eat, that also happen to be nutritionally sound. So all you have to do is reach in the pantry or fridge for the ingredients to make a quick dish—in 15 minutes (and sometimes less)!

This book is mostly for people who have diabetes, but it's also for people who simply want to eat healthier without a lot of effort. It contains everyday, real food and familiar-sounding (and tasting) recipes that can be prepared in 15 minutes flat.

What can you cook in 15 minutes? A lot! By using just a few ingredients, convenience items—such as salsa, pre-cut veggies, pre-cooked meats, poultry—and taking advantage of the tremendous choices in the grocer's freezer section, healthy dishes can be made in a fraction of the time.

This book contains more than 200 recipes, covering everything from appetizers and beverages to desserts. And because the time is so short, the ingredient list has to be short. So you save time on shopping, money, storage, prepping, and cleanup!

So what are you waiting for? All you need is...15 minutes!

Enjoy!

—N.H.

ACKNOWLEDGMENTS

Thanks to Robert Anthony, my editor and idea-bouncer-off-er, for being there when I needed you, for calling on me when you needed me, and for all the times between. You make working with the giant organization of the American Diabetes Association personable and an absolute pleasure!

To my assistants, Monica Davis, Tracy Woodham, Wes Shepherd, and Nicholas Norman...whew, we did it...together. Thanks for tasting, testing, shopping, and cleaning up—over and over again!

SOMETHING TO THINK ABOUT

In 15 minutes, you can call for pizza delivery or you can stand in a long fast-food line. But think about this:

It takes that long (and sometimes longer) to order it, wait for it, and pay a lot for it! So why not take those same 15 minutes and enjoy healthier, cheaper, and more flavorful dishes that make you feel better all the way around? It's your choice.

It's something to think about!

INTRODUCTION

10 SIMPLE SUGGESTIONS FOR ENJOYING THESE RECIPES EVEN MORE

1. **Stock Up.** Stock up on enough ingredients to make at least three or four meals, and store them in your freezer, refrigerator, and pantry so you'll never be lost for meal ideas. When you keep a few basics on hand, you'll be surprised at the peace of mind it brings you, which cuts down on stress, lapses in willpower, and dollars!

2. **Use Your Supermarket.**

   - **Produce Aisle:** Take advantage of the prepared ingredients in the supermarket produce section, such as bagged lettuce mixes, greens, baby carrots, and other prepped fruits and vegetables, including pre-chopped items on the salad bar—especially when you really need to shave time off your "already-quick" recipes.
   - **Freezer Section:** This section is really bulging with tons of new choices that can speed things up in the kitchen, including frozen cooked brown rice.
   - **Buy One, Get One Free:** Very often, supermarkets run specials on items throughout the store; this is a good time to grab lean cuts of meat. Keep in mind that sale items are only a bargain if you are actually going to use them. Stock up and store them in your freezer to keep on hand, but wrap them in individual

serving sizes so you can thaw out only what you need instead of the whole package.

3. **Bring Home the Chicken.** On days you need a little extra help, pick up a couple of rotisserie chickens. Yes, a couple of chickens so you can save steps. Enjoy a roast chicken one night and debone the rest and freeze it. That way you can have it ready when you need it for those quick sandwich, soup, salad, and casserole recipes that call for cooked chicken. Just don't forget to remove the skin first!

4. **Pull It Out.** I've said this in every book that I've written, but it is one of the most important steps in cooking. Before you start a recipe, read through it first, then put everything on the counter and prep the items as written in the ingredient list before starting the directions. Doing this makes a tremendous difference in the timing and end results of the recipe.

5. **Triple It.** When making salad dressings from this book, triple or even quadruple the recipe so you can keep it in the fridge for later uses (as you would with a bottle of store-bought dressing). Also, it's helpful to have several types of salad dressing on hand to keep your salad-making interesting and easy. Try drizzling a different dressing than usual over sliced cucumbers and tomatoes, or use salad dressings instead of mayonnaise on sandwiches or burgers.

6. **Substitute with Fruits and Veggies.** Be creative, and keep in mind that you can use fruits or veggies with any of the dips that are for crackers, chips, or breads.

7. **Change the Look.** Be creative with your veggie dippers; for example, don't limit yourself to the vegetable choices in the ingredient list. You can change them up and use blanched asparagus spears or whole green beans. Or you can do something as simple as cutting a vegetable in a

more interesting manner, such as cutting yellow squash or cucumber diagonally instead of rounds.

8. **Changes with Color and Crunch.** Keep variety in mind when you're planning your salads and sandwiches. Color and texture are important factors. Try adding peeled zucchini strips or crunchy red cabbage to your salads. Something as simple as changing from yellow onions to red onions, or from green bell peppers to yellow, can brighten up a salad or sandwich instantly.

9. **Build It Bigger.** If you want to give your salad more body and character, add pre-sliced mushrooms, broccoli florets, a handful of green peas, or a few garbanzo beans. And don't underestimate the power of fresh herbs, such as basil, cilantro, and even parsley. Herbs add an explosion of flavor to every bite.

And finally...

10. **List It.** While flipping through the recipes, you might want to make a list of the recipes that look like they may bring comfort to you. (I can't function without lists, even though I tend to lose them.) Everybody has their own definition of what brings them comfort. To me, every day requires a different comfort; if you're the same, write down the titles (with the page numbers) of the recipes that hit your "comfort" moods. You might even want to take it a step further and jot down "special occasion" lists, such as a list of recipes you'd like to serve company. Or maybe a list for fun weeknight recipes. Or maybe one for the kids or grandkids. No matter what the occasion, with a list, all you have to do is glance and go!

BREAKFASTS

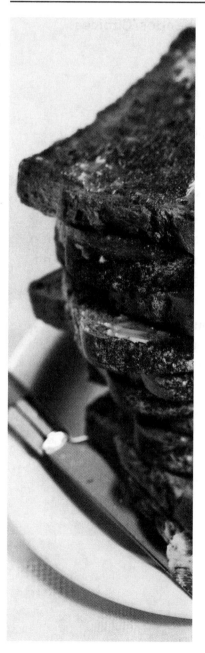

HOT AND STEAMING SWEET PLUM OATMEAL

Serves: 4 • Serving Size: 3/4 cup

4	cups water
2	cups quick-cooking oats
20	orange essence dried plums, chopped
2	tablespoons reduced-fat margarine
1 1/2	teaspoons ground cinnamon
2	tablespoons pourable brown sugar substitute
1	teaspoon vanilla, or 1/2 teaspoon vanilla, butter, and nut flavoring

1. In a medium saucepan, bring water to boil over high heat and stir in oats and plums. Reduce heat and simmer 1 minute, stirring frequently.

2. Remove from heat, stir in remaining ingredients, cover tightly, and let stand 5 minutes to absorb flavors and thicken slightly.

Exchanges/Choices

2 Starch
1 1/2 Fruit
1 Fat

Calories	290
Calories from Fat	45
Total Fat	5.0 g
Saturated Fat	1.2 g
Trans Fat	0.0 g
Cholesterol	0 mg
Sodium	60 mg
Total Carbohydrate	54 g
Dietary Fiber	8 g
Sugars	14 g
Protein	6 g

BANANA-SPICED OATMEAL

Serves: 4 • Serving Size: 1 cup

Exchanges/Choices

1 1/2 Starch
1 Fruit
1 Fat

Calories	215	
Calories from Fat	45	
Total Fat	5.0	g
Saturated Fat	1.2	g
Trans Fat	0.0	g
Cholesterol	0	mg
Sodium	120	mg
Total Carbohydrate	38	g
Dietary Fiber	5	g
Sugars	10	g
Protein	5	g

3	cups water
1 1/2	cups quick-cooking oats
2	ripe medium bananas, peeled and diced
3 to 4	tablespoons pourable sugar substitute
2	teaspoons ground cinnamon
1/4	teaspoon ground nutmeg
1/8	teaspoon salt
1 1/2	tablespoons reduced-fat margarine
1	tablespoon vanilla extract

1. Bring water to a boil in a large saucepan. Stir in the oats, return just to a boil, reduce heat and simmer, uncovered, 1 minute.

2. Remove from heat, add remaining ingredients, cover, and let stand 5 minutes to absorb flavors.

ZESTY NEW DAY CEREAL

Serves 8 • Serving Size: 3/4 cup cereal and 1/2 cup milk

1/2 cup pecan pieces
4 cups oatmeal squares with cinnamon cereal
1 cup high-fiber, thread-style cereal
1/2 cup dried cherries
1 teaspoon grated orange zest
1 teaspoon ground cinnamon
4 cups fat-free milk

1. Place a large nonstick skillet over medium-high heat. Cook the pecans 2 minutes or until fragrant and beginning to lightly brown, stirring frequently. Set aside on separate plate.

2. Combine all ingredients in a gallon-size resealable plastic bag. Seal tightly and shake until well blended. Serve in bowls and pour 1/2 cup fat-free milk over each serving of cereal.

3. Store remaining cereal mixture in sealed bag in pantry.

Values do not include milk

Exchanges/Choices

2 Starch
1/2 Fruit
1 Fat

Calories	210	
Calories from Fat	65	
Total Fat	7.0	g
Saturated Fat	0.7	g
Trans Fat	0.0	g
Cholesterol	0	mg
Sodium	160	mg
Total Carbohydrate	39	g
Dietary Fiber	7	g
Sugars	0	g
Protein	4	g

Cook's Note

This recipe also makes a great snack or trail mix!

FRUIT AND PEANUT BUTTER CINNAMON TOAST

Serves: 4 • Serving Size: 1 sandwich

Exchanges/Choices

1 Starch
1 Fruit
1 Med-Fat Meat

Calories	225	
Calories from Fat	65	
Total Fat	7.0	g
Saturated Fat	1.3	g
Trans Fat	0.0	g
Cholesterol	0	mg
Sodium	185	mg
Total Carbohydrate	33	g
Dietary Fiber	4	g
Sugars	15	g
Protein	8	g

1/4 cup reduced-fat peanut butter
4 slices cinnamon raisin whole-wheat bread, toasted
1 medium banana, peeled and sliced
1/2 cup fresh or frozen, unsweetened, thawed blueberries
2 teaspoons honey

1. Spread equal amounts peanut butter on each bread slice, then top with equal amounts banana and berries. Drizzle honey evenly over all.

MANGO AND CHEESECAKE SPREAD ON CINNAMON ENGLISH MUFFINS

Serves 4 • Serving Size: 2 muffin halves

1/2 cup fat-free cream cheese

2 tablespoons fat-free milk

1 teaspoon vanilla

2 teaspoons pourable sugar substitute

4 cinnamon raisin English muffins (preferably whole wheat), halved and lightly toasted

1 cup diced mango or nectarine

1. Combine the cream cheese, milk, vanilla, and sugar substitute in a small microwave-safe bowl. Cook on HIGH setting 15 seconds or until cream cheese is softened. Stir until well blended.

2. Spread equal amounts of the cream cheese mixture evenly over each muffin half. Top with equal amounts of the fruit.

Exchanges/Choices

2 Starch

1/2 Fruit

Calories	200
Calories from Fat	10
Total Fat	1.0 g
Saturated Fat	0.3 g
Trans Fat	0.0 g
Cholesterol	5 mg
Sodium	405 mg
Total Carbohydrate	37 g
Dietary Fiber	2 g
Sugars	16 g
Protein	9 g

MINI BAGELS WITH SMOKED SALMON

Serves: 4 • Serving Size: 2 bagel halves

Exchanges/Choices

2 Starch

1 Lean Meat

Calories	180
Calories from Fat	15
Total Fat	1.5 g
Saturated Fat	0.3 g
Trans Fat	N/A
Cholesterol	10 mg
Sodium	600 mg
Total Carbohydrate	28 g
Dietary Fiber	3 g
Sugars	6 g
Protein	14 g

4 whole-wheat mini bagels, halved

4 ounces fat-free cream cheese

2 teaspoons capers (preferably small variety), rinsed and drained

1/2 cup finely chopped tomatoes

3 ounces smoked salmon, thinly sliced and chopped

1 teaspoon dried dill weed

1. Place bagels on a baking sheet under the broiler (not preheated). Turn on broiler and toast 1 to 2 minutes or until golden.

2. Remove from heat and spread bagels evenly with the cream cheese. Top with the capers, tomatoes, salmon, and dill weed.

MORNING WAFFLES WITH VANILLA BLACKBERRIES

Serves: 6 • Serving Size: 1 waffle, about 1/2 cup blackberry mixture, and 1/4 cup yogurt

1	pound frozen unsweetened blackberries, thawed
3	tablespoons sugar
1/2	teaspoon vanilla
1/2	teaspoon grated lemon zest
6	frozen whole-grain waffles
1 1/2	cups vanilla yogurt with mainly low-calorie sweeteners

1. In a medium bowl, combine blackberries, sugar, vanilla, and lemon zest and set aside.

2. Toast waffles, place on individual dinner plates, spoon equal amounts of the blackberry mixture on each, and top with equal amounts of the yogurt.

Exchanges/Choices

1 Starch
1 Fruit
1/2 Fat-Free Milk
1/2 Fat

Calories	205	
Calories from Fat	45	
Total Fat	5.0	g
Saturated Fat	1.3	g
Trans Fat	0	g
Cholesterol	40	mg
Sodium	220	mg
Total Carbohydrate	36	g
Dietary Fiber	5	g
Sugars	21	g
Protein	6	g

CRISPY BREAKFAST PITA ROUNDS

Serves: 4 • Serving Size: 1 pita round

Exchanges/Choices

1 1/2 Starch
1/2 Fruit
1 Med-Fat Meat

Calories	240	
Calories from Fat	65	
Total Fat	7.0	g
Saturated Fat	3.0	g
Trans Fat	0.0	g
Cholesterol	15	mg
Sodium	495	mg
Total Carbohydrate	31	g
Dietary Fiber	3	g
Sugars	12	g
Protein	14	g

2 6-inch pita rounds
2 veggie breakfast patties, finely chopped
1/4 cup finely chopped green bell pepper
1 plum tomato, finely chopped
1/4 cup finely chopped green onion
1/4 teaspoon dried red pepper flakes, optional
3/4 cup shredded reduced-fat sharp cheddar or part-skim mozzarella cheese
1 medium cantaloupe, cut into 4 wedges

1. Preheat oven to 475°F.

2. Using a sharp knife, cut pita rounds in half creating four rounds total. Place on a baking sheet. In the order listed, top each round with equal amounts of the remaining ingredients, except the cantaloupe.

3. Bake 5 minutes or until cheese melts. Serve with cantaloupe wedges

ENGLISH MUFFINS WITH APRICOT-GINGER SPREAD

Serves: 4 • Serving Size: 2 muffin halves and spread

3 tablespoons reduced-fat margarine
1/4 cup apricot 100% fruit spread
1 teaspoon grated ginger
1 teaspoon honey
4 whole-wheat English muffins, halved

1. In a small mixing bowl, combine all ingredients except muffins and stir to blend. The mixture will be lumpy.

2. Toast muffins and spread equal amounts of the mixture on each muffin half. The spread will melt into the muffins.

Exchanges/Choices

2 Starch
1/2 Carbohydrate
1/2 Fat

Calories	215
Calories from Fat	45
Total Fat	5.0 g
Saturated Fat	1.3 g
Trans Fat	0.0 g
Cholesterol	0 mg
Sodium	380 mg
Total Carbohydrate	38 g
Dietary Fiber	5 g
Sugars	15 g
Protein	6 g

Cook's Note
This breakfast item also makes a great snack later in the day!

ON-THE-RUN BREAKFAST GRAHAM PILE UPS

Serves: 4 • Serving Size: 1 pile up

Exchanges/Choices

1/2 Fat-Free Milk
2 1/2 Carbohydrate
1 High-Fat Meat

Calories	325
Calories from Fat	110
Total Fat	12.0 g
Saturated Fat	2.2 g
Trans Fat	0.0 g
Cholesterol	0 mg
Sodium	310 mg
Total Carbohydrate	42 g
Dietary Fiber	3 g
Sugars	22 g
Protein	13 g

1/2 cup reduced-fat peanut butter
4 low-fat cinnamon graham crackers (about 2 inches by 5 inches each)
3 tablespoons apple butter
1 cup diced apples (preferably Granny Smith variety)
2 cups fat-free milk

1. Spread equal amounts of the peanut butter on each of the graham crackers. Lightly spoon the apple butter over all. Top with the apples and serve each with 4 ounces of milk.

Cook's Note

If you want two smaller pile ups instead of one large one, break each cracker in half before topping with remaining ingredients.

THE STACKED SCRAMBLE

Serves: 4 • Serving Size: 1/4 recipe

2	cups egg substitute
1/3	cup fat-free evaporated milk
2	medium tomatoes, seeded and chopped
1/2	medium green bell pepper, finely chopped
1/4	cup chopped cilantro or parsley leaves
1/8	teaspoon cayenne pepper, optional
2/3	cup shredded reduced-fat sharp cheddar cheese

1. Preheat broiler.

2. In a medium mixing bowl, combine egg substitute and milk; stir to blend.

3. Place a large ovenproof skillet over medium heat until hot. Coat skillet with cooking spray, add eggs, and cook 2 minutes, lifting cooked portion up with a spatula to allow uncooked portion to flow underneath.

4. Remove skillet from heat and sprinkle eggs evenly with remaining ingredients in the order given. Broil 2 minutes or until cheese melts. Salt and pepper to taste.

Exchanges/Choices

1/2 Carbohydrate
3 Lean Meat

Calories	150	
Calories from Fat	35	
Total Fat	4.0	g
Saturated Fat	2.4	g
Trans Fat	0.0	g
Cholesterol	15	mg
Sodium	415	mg
Total Carbohydrate	9	g
Dietary Fiber	1	g
Sugars	6	g
Protein	19	g

GARDEN FRESH SPINACH OMELET

Serves: 4 • Serving Size: 1/2 omelet

Exchanges/Choices

1/2 Carbohydrate
1 Med-Fat Meat

Calories	120
Calories from Fat	25
Total Fat	3.0 g
Saturated Fat	1.8 g
Trans Fat	0.0 g
Cholesterol	10 mg
Sodium	415 mg
Total Carbohydrate	5 g
Dietary Fiber	1 g
Sugars	3 g
Protein	17 g

2 cups egg substitute
1/4 cup fat-free milk
2 cups (2 ounces total) loosely packed baby spinach
1 4-ounce container sliced pimiento, drained
1/2 teaspoon dried thyme leaves
1/4 teaspoon dried red pepper flakes
1/2 cup shredded reduced-fat sharp cheddar cheese

1. Preheat oven 200°F. Combine the eggs and milk in a medium bowl and stir until well blended

2. Place a small nonstick skillet over medium heat until hot. Coat skillet with cooking spray and then pour 1/2 of the egg mixture into skillet. Cook over medium heat 5 to 6 minutes. As eggs begin to set, gently lift edge of omelet with spatula and tilt skillet so uncooked portion flows underneath.

3. When egg mixture is set, spoon 1/2 of the spinach, pimiento, thyme, pepper flakes, and cheese over half of omelet. Loosen omelet with spatula and fold over in half. Slide omelet onto serving plate and place in oven to keep warm. Repeat with remaining ingredients to make second omelet.

4. To serve, cut each omelet in half and place on four dinner plates. Lightly salt and pepper to taste, if desired.

SKILLET SWISS CORN SCRAMBLE

Serves: 4 • Serving Size: 1 cup

2 cups egg substitute

3/4 cup diced extra-lean ham

1 cup frozen corn kernels, thawed

1/4 cup fat-free milk

1 teaspoon dried thyme leaves

3 ounces (4 slices) thin-sliced reduced-fat Swiss cheese

1/4 cup finely chopped green onion or parsley

1. Combine the eggs, ham, corn, milk, and thyme in a medium bowl.

2. Place a large nonstick skillet over medium heat until hot. Lightly coat with cooking spray, cook the egg mixture 2 to 3 minutes, lifting cooked portion up with a spatula to allow uncooked portion to flow underneath.

3. Remove skillet from heat and sprinkle eggs evenly with the cheese and onions. Sprinkle with black pepper, if desired. Cover and let stand 2 minutes to allow flavors to absorb and cheese to melt.

Exchanges/Choices

1 Starch
3 Lean Meat

Calories	190	
Calories from Fat	45	
Total Fat	5.0	g
Saturated Fat	2.3	g
Trans Fat	0.0	g
Cholesterol	25	mg
Sodium	595	mg
Total Carbohydrate	12	g
Dietary Fiber	1	g
Sugars	5	g
Protein	26	g

BREAKWICHES

Serves: 4 • Serving Size: 1 sandwich

Exchanges/Choices
1 1/2 Starch
2 Lean Meat
1 Fat

Calories	240	
Calories from Fat	80	
Total Fat	9.0	g
Saturated Fat	2.1	g
Trans Fat	0.0	g
Cholesterol	30	mg
Sodium	1035	mg
Total Carbohydrate	25	g
Dietary Fiber	6	g
Sugars	4	g
Protein	19	g

1/4 cup reduced-fat mayonnaise
2 teaspoons Dijon mustard
8 slices reduced-calorie whole-wheat bread, lightly toasted
1 cup egg substitute
1 cup diced extra-lean ham
1/4 cup finely chopped green onions
1/4 cup shredded reduced-fat sharp cheddar cheese

1. Stir together the mayonnaise with the mustard in a small bowl. Spread equal amounts on four of the bread slices.

2. Place a large nonstick skillet over medium heat. Lightly coat skillet with cooking spray, cook the eggs 1 to 2 minutes, lifting cooked portion up with a spatula to allow uncooked portion to flow underneath. Sprinkle evenly with the ham, onions, and cheese. Remove from heat. Spoon equal amounts on four of the bread slices and top with the remaining bread slices. Press down lightly to allow ingredients to hold together.

GRILLED CHEESE BREAKFAST PANINI

Serves: 4 • Serving Size: 1 sandwich

1	cup egg substitute
3/4	cup shredded reduced-fat mozzarella cheese
1	large tomato, cut into 8 slices
16	fresh basil leaves
16	turkey pepperoni slices, halved (optional)
1/2	of a 16-ounce loaf whole-wheat or multigrain Italian bread, cut into 8 slices

1. Place a large nonstick skillet over medium heat. Lightly coat skillet with cooking spray, cook the eggs, about 1 to 2 minutes, lifting cooked portion up with a spatula to allow uncooked portion to flow underneath. Remove eggs from skillet and set aside on separate plate.

2. Lightly coat both sides of each bread slice with cooking spray. Top four bread slices with equal amounts cheese, tomato, basil, pepperoni, and scrambled eggs. Top with remaining bread slices. Press down lightly to allow ingredients to hold together.

3. Wipe skillet clean with a damp paper towel, lightly coat with cooking spray and place over medium heat. Cook sandwiches 3 minutes on each side, or until golden on the bottom, pressing down frequently with a flat spatula to flatten slightly and give the appearance of a panini.

Exchanges/Choices

2 Starch
2 Lean Meat

Calories	235
Calories from Fat	45
Total Fat	5.0 g
Saturated Fat	1.9 g
Trans Fat	0.5 g
Cholesterol	5 mg
Sodium	530 mg
Total Carbohydrate	27 g
Dietary Fiber	4 g
Sugars	5 g
Protein	20 g

AVOCADO AND BLACK BEAN EARLY MORNING BURRITOS

Serves: 4 • Serving Size: 1 burrito

Exchanges/Choices

2 Starch
1 Vegetable
2 Lean Meat
1 Fat

Calories	320
Calories from Fat	80
Total Fat	9.0 g
Saturated Fat	1.4 g
Trans Fat	0.0 g
Cholesterol	5 mg
Sodium	740 mg
Total Carbohydrate	42 g
Dietary Fiber	10 g
Sugars	4 g
Protein	21 g

1 ripe medium avocado, peeled, pitted, and diced
1/2 of a 15.5-ounce can black beans, rinsed and drained
2 medium limes
1/2 teaspoon ground cumin
4 whole-wheat flour tortillas
2 cups egg substitute
1/2 cup mild picante sauce
1/2 cup fat-free sour cream
2 tablespoons chopped cilantro

1. Combine avocado, beans, the juice of one of the limes, and cumin in a medium bowl. Toss gently and set aside.

2. Heat tortillas according to microwave directions on package.

3. Place a large nonstick skillet over medium heat until hot. Lightly coat with cooking spray, cook the eggs 2 minutes, lifting cooked portion up with a spatula to allow uncooked portion to flow underneath.

4. Remove skillet from heat. Place a tortilla on each of the four dinner plates. In the center of each tortilla, spoon equal amounts of the eggs and top with the picante sauce, sour cream, avocado mixture, and cilantro. Serve with the remaining lime cut in wedges.

Cook's Note

This dish can be served with knives and forks for open-faced burritos or folded together at the edges for wrapped burritos.

FRENCH TOAST WITH APPLE BUTTER & PEARS

Serves: 4 • Serving Size: 1 French toast with toppings

1/4 cup (1 ounce) chopped pecans
1 cup egg substitute
4 slices reduced-calorie whole-wheat bread
1 teaspoon canola oil
1/4 cup apple butter
1 cup fat-free vanilla yogurt with mainly low-calorie sweeteners
1 cup chopped ripe pears

1. Place a large nonstick skillet over medium-high heat. Cook the pecans 2 minutes or until fragrant and beginning to lightly brown, stirring frequently. Set aside on separate plate.

2. Place the bread slices in a large pan, such as a 13-inch by 9-inch baking pan. Pour the egg substitute over all and turn the bread slices over several times to coat well.

3. Heat the oil in the skillet over medium-high heat. Tilt the skillet to coat bottom lightly. Cook the bread 3 minutes, turn, and cook 2 minutes longer or until golden brown on the bottom.

4. Place on four individual dinner plates, top each with 1 tablespoon of the apple butter, 1/4 cup yogurt, and 1/4 cup pears.

Exchanges/Choices

1/2 Fat-Free Milk
1 1/2 Carbohydrate
1 Lean Meat
1/2 Fat

Calories	215
Calories from Fat	65
Total Fat	7.0 g
Saturated Fat	0.7 g
Trans Fat	0.0 g
Cholesterol	0 mg
Sodium	260 mg
Total Carbohydrate	30 g
Dietary Fiber	5 g
Sugars	15 g
Protein	11 g

SMOKED SAUSAGE AND CHEDDAR-TOPPED GRITS

Serves: 4 • Serving Size: 1/2 cup grits, 2 tablespoons cheese, and 1/3 cup sausage mixture

Exchanges/Choices

1 1/2 Starch
1 Med-Fat Meat
1/2 Fat

Calories	215
Calories from Fat	70
Total Fat	8.0 g
Saturated Fat	3.3 g
Trans Fat	0.0 g
Cholesterol	30 mg
Sodium	600 mg
Total Carbohydrate	24 g
Dietary Fiber	1 g
Sugars	5 g
Protein	12 g

2 1/4 cups water
1/2 cup dry quick-cooking grits
1 cup finely chopped green bell pepper
8 ounces diced smoked turkey sausage
1 teaspoon Worcestershire sauce
1/2 cup shredded reduced-fat sharp cheddar cheese

1. Bring 2 cups of the water to a boil in a medium saucepan over high heat. Stir in grits, return to a boil, reduce heat, cover tightly, and simmer 5 minutes or until liquid is absorbed.

2. Meanwhile, place a large nonstick skillet over medium-high heat until hot. Coat skillet with cooking spray, add peppers, coat with cooking spray, cook 4 minutes or until beginning to lightly brown on edges. Add sausage, coat lightly with cooking spray, and cook 3 minutes or until beginning to lightly brown on edges. Add the remaining 1/4 cup water and the Worcestershire sauce and cook 15 seconds, stirring constantly.

3. Place equal amounts of grits on four dinner plates, sprinkle evenly with the cheese, and spoon equal amounts of the sausage mixture on top.

BREAKFAST TURKEY SAUSAGE AND CINNAMON APPLES

Serves: 4 • Serving Size: 2 links and 1/2 cup apple mixture

8 lean breakfast turkey sausage links

3 (12 ounces total) medium red apples, halved, cored, and sliced

2 tablespoons raisins

1/2 teaspoon ground cinnamon

1 tablespoon reduced-fat margarine

2 teaspoons honey

1. Place a large nonstick skillet over medium-high heat until hot. Coat skillet with cooking spray, add the sausage, and cook 8 minutes or until no longer pink in center, turning frequently. Remove from skillet and set aside.

2. Coat skillet with cooking spray, add the apples, raisins, cinnamon, and margarine, and cook 1 minute, stirring gently, yet constantly, using two utensils as you would for a stir fry.

3. Remove from heat, add the sausage, and drizzle honey over all. Toss gently, about 15 seconds or until coated. Cover and let stand 3 minutes to absorb flavors.

Exchanges/Choices

1 Fruit
2 Med-Fat Meat

Calories	195
Calories from Fat	70
Total Fat	8.0 g
Saturated Fat	2.4 g
Trans Fat	0.0 g
Cholesterol	45 mg
Sodium	495 mg
Total Carbohydrate	19 g
Dietary Fiber	2 g
Sugars	14 g
Protein	13 g

DARK-SAUCED PORK CHOPS

Serves: 4 • Serving Size: 3 ounces pork

Exchanges/Choices

3 Lean Meat
1/2 Fat

Calories	155
Calories from Fat	65
Total Fat	7.0 g
Saturated Fat	2.3 g
Trans Fat	0.0 g
Cholesterol	60 mg
Sodium	50 mg
Total Carbohydrate	1 g
Dietary Fiber	0 g
Sugars	0 g
Protein	21 g

1/2 teaspoon chili powder
1/4 teaspoon garlic powder
1 teaspoon instant coffee granules
4 (about 1 1/4 pounds total) thin lean pork chops with bone in
1 teaspoon olive oil
1/2 cup water
2 teaspoons balsamic vinegar

1. Combine the chili powder, garlic powder, and coffee granules in a small bowl. Sprinkle evenly over both sides of the pork, pressing down with fingertips to adhere.

2. Heat the oil in a large nonstick skillet over medium-high heat. Cook the pork 3 minutes on each side or until barely pink in center. Set aside on separate plate.

3. Add the water and vinegar to the pan residue in skillet. Bring to a boil over medium-high heat and boil 3 minutes or until reduced to 2 tablespoons, scraping bottom and sides. Spoon evenly over the pork and lightly season with salt and pepper, if desired.

BORDER BREAKFAST STEAKS WITH CILANTRO

Serves: 4 • Serving Size: 1/4 recipe

1	teaspoon chili powder
1/4	teaspoon ground cumin
1/4	teaspoon onion powder
1	pound trimmed thin round steak, cut into four pieces
1/4	cup water
1	medium tomato, diced
1/4	cup chopped cilantro
1	medium lime, cut in wedges
1/4	cup fat-free sour cream (optional)

1. Combine the chili powder, cumin, and onion powder in a small bowl. Sprinkle evenly over both sides of the beef, pressing down lightly with fingertips to adhere.

2. Place a large nonstick skillet over medium-high heat until hot. Coat lightly with cooking spray, cook the beef 2 minutes, turn, and cook 1 minute or until very pink in center. Place on serving platter and set aside.

3. Add the water and tomatoes to pan residue in skillet over medium-high heat and cook 2 minutes or until reduced slightly, scraping bottom and sides of skillet. Pour evenly over the beef. Season lightly with salt and pepper, if desired. Sprinkle evenly with the cilantro. Serve with lime wedges and top with sour cream, if desired.

Exchanges/Choices

4 Lean Meat

Calories	165
Calories from Fat	55
Total Fat	6.0 g
Saturated Fat	2.0 g
Trans Fat	0.1 g
Cholesterol	75 mg
Sodium	45 mg
Total Carbohydrate	2 g
Dietary Fiber	1 g
Sugars	1 g
Protein	25 g

BREAKFAST BLAST IN A GLASS

Serves: 4 • Serving Size: 1 cup

Exchanges/Choices

1 Fruit
1 Fat-Free Milk

Calories	155
Calories from Fat	15
Total Fat	1.5 g
Saturated Fat	1.0 g
Trans Fat	0.0 g
Cholesterol	10 mg
Sodium	70 mg
Total Carbohydrate	31 g
Dietary Fiber	2 g
Sugars	26 g
Protein	6 g

1 small banana, peeled and sliced
2 cups low-fat vanilla yogurt with mainly low-calorie sweeteners
2 cups frozen unsweetened peaches, slightly thawed

1. Place ingredients in a blender, secure with lid, and blend until smooth.

ENERGY ON-THE-GO SMOOTHIES

Serves: 2 • Serving Size: 1 1/2 cups

2 cups (16 ounces) nonfat vanilla yogurt with mainly low-calorie sweeteners

1 ripe medium banana, peeled

2 tablespoons reduced-fat peanut butter

1/2 teaspoon ground cinnamon

1 teaspoon vanilla

1 cup ice cubes

1. Combine all ingredients in a blender, secure with lid, and puree until smooth. Pour into 2 tall glasses.

Exchanges/Choices

1 Fruit

1 Fat-Free Milk

1 Carbohydrate

1 Fat

Calories	265
Calories from Fat	55
Total Fat	6.0 g
Saturated Fat	1.3 g
Trans Fat	0.0 g
Cholesterol	5 mg
Sodium	185 mg
Total Carbohydrate	44 g
Dietary Fiber	3 g
Sugars	25 g
Protein	11 g

Cook's Note

To serve four, double the recipe above, but puree in two batches.

START-THE-DAY BERRY PARFAIT

Serves: 4 • Serving Size: 1 parfait

Exchanges/Choices

1 Starch
2 Fruit
1 Fat-Free Milk

Calories	290
Calories from Fat	25
Total Fat	3.0 g
Saturated Fat	1.3 g
Trans Fat	0.0 g
Cholesterol	10 mg
Sodium	130 mg
Total Carbohydrate	61 g
Dietary Fiber	5 g
Sugars	23 g
Protein	8 g

1 1/2 cups fresh or frozen, thawed unsweetened blueberries
1/4 cup raspberry 100% fruit spread
2 1/2 cups sliced fresh strawberries
2 teaspoons grated orange zest
1 teaspoon grated ginger
1/4 teaspoon ground cinnamon
2 cups low-fat vanilla yogurt with mainly low-calorie sweeteners
1 cup low-fat granola

1. Place fruit spread in a small microwave-safe bowl and microwave on HIGH setting 5 to 10 seconds or until fruit spread has melted slightly.

2. In a medium bowl, combine strawberries, blueberries, grated orange zest, ginger, fruit spread, and cinnamon.

3. Spoon 1/4 cup yogurt in the bottom of four clear glasses, wine goblets, or dessert bowls. Top with 1/2 cup fruit mixture, then 2 tablespoons granola. Repeat all layers once.

Cook's Note

If using frozen blueberries, place in a colander and run under cold water 10 to 15 seconds to thaw quickly, but still keep firm. Drain on paper towels and set aside.

CREAMY LEMON AND PINEAPPLE BUSY DAY PARFAITS

Serves: 4 • Serving Size: about 1 1/2 cups

2 ounces (1/2 cup) sliced almonds

3 tablespoons apricot 100% fruit spread

1 8-ounce can pineapple tidbits in its own juice, drained

4 6-ounce containers fat-free lemon or lime yogurt with mainly low-calorie sweeteners

1 1/3 cups (about 3 ounces) high-fiber cluster-style cereal

1 cup diced strawberries

1. Place a large nonstick skillet over medium-high heat. Cook the almonds 2 minutes or until fragrant and beginning to lightly brown, stirring frequently. Set aside on separate plate.

2. Spoon the fruit spread into a medium microwave-safe bowl and cook on high setting 15 seconds until slightly melted. Stir in the pineapple. Spoon equal amounts in each of four parfait dishes or wine goblets. Top with the yogurt, cereal, strawberries, and the almonds.

Exchanges/Choices

1 Starch
1 Fruit
1 Fat-Free Milk
1 Fat

Calories	285
Calories from Fat	70
Total Fat	8.0 g
Saturated Fat	0.8 g
Trans Fat	0.0 g
Cholesterol	5 mg
Sodium	195 mg
Total Carbohydrate	49 g
Dietary Fiber	7 g
Sugars	27 g
Protein	10 g

ANY MORNING, ANY TIME SUNDAES

Serves: 4 • Serving Size: about 1 cup

Exchanges/Choices

2 1/2 Carbohydrate

Calories	185
Calories from Fat	20
Total Fat	2.0 g
Saturated Fat	0.8 g
Trans Fat	0.0 g
Cholesterol	10 mg
Sodium	85 mg
Total Carbohydrate	37 g
Dietary Fiber	3 g
Sugars	26 g
Protein	6 g

2 cups fat-free vanilla frozen yogurt
2 cups sliced strawberries
1/2 cup low-fat granola
4 teaspoons mini chocolate chips

1. Spoon 1/2 cup of yogurt into each of four dessert bowls. Top each with 1/2 cup strawberries, 2 tablespoons granola, and 1 teaspoon chocolate chips.

LUNCHES

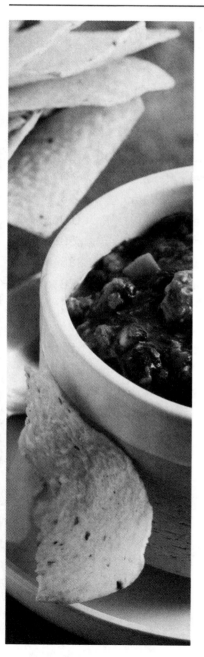

OVERSTUFFED AND CRUNCHY TURKEY VEGGIE SUBS

Serves: 4 • Serving Size: 1 sandwich

8 ounces multigrain Italian bread, cut in half lengthwise and cut in fourths crosswise

4 tomato slices, halved

3 slices light provolone cheese, quartered

4 ounces deli-sliced oven-roasted turkey

2 cups loosely packed shredded lettuce

2 ounces pepperoncinis, sliced

1 tablespoon extra virgin olive oil

1 teaspoon cider vinegar

1. Place bottom half of bread on a clean work surface, then place equal amounts on top in the following order: tomatoes, three pieces of the quartered cheese, turkey, lettuce, and pepperoncinis.

2. Combine the oil and vinegar in a small bowl and stir until well blended. Spoon 1 teaspoon of the mixture evenly over each serving. Top with remaining bread halves and press down firmly to hold together better.

Exchanges/Choices

2 Starch
2 Lean Meat
1/2 Fat

Calories	270	
Calories from Fat	80	
Total Fat	9.0	g
Saturated Fat	2.5	g
Trans Fat	0.0	g
Cholesterol	30	mg
Sodium	385	mg
Total Carbohydrate	28	g
Dietary Fiber	5	g
Sugars	6	g
Protein	20	g

HAM AND SWISS SCALLION QUESADILLAS

Serves: 4 • Serving Size: 2 quesadilla wedges

Exchanges/Choices

2 Starch
1 Fruit
2 Med-Fat Meat

Calories	360
Calories from Fat	100
Total Fat	11.0 g
Saturated Fat	3.5 g
Trans Fat	0.0 g
Cholesterol	20 mg
Sodium	655 mg
Total Carbohydrate	52 g
Dietary Fiber	6 g
Sugars	12 g
Protein	17 g

3/4 cup reduced-fat Swiss cheese, torn in small pieces
4 10-inch flour tortillas
2 ounces extra-lean ham, thinly sliced and chopped
1/2 medium red bell pepper, finely chopped
1/2 cup finely chopped green onion
4 cups fresh sliced strawberries

1. Preheat oven to warm. Place 1/4 of the cheese on 1/2 of each tortilla.

2. Top each cheese portion with 1/2 ounce ham, 2 tablespoons bell pepper, and 2 tablespoons onion. Fold over tortillas and press down gently to make them adhere.

3. Place a large nonstick skillet over medium heat until hot. Coat both sides of two tortillas with cooking spray and place in skillet. Cook 2 minutes, turn, and cook 1 to 2 minutes longer or until cheese has melted and tortillas are golden.

4. Remove from heat and place in oven to keep warm. Repeat with remaining two tortillas. Using a serrated knife, cut tortillas in half, beginning on the folded side for easier cutting. Serve strawberries on the side.

CHEESY HAM AND GREEN ONION MELT

Serves: 4 • Serving Size: 1 sandwich

1/3 cup finely diced lean ham

1/2 cup finely chopped green onions

1/2 cup grated reduced-fat sharp cheddar cheese

3 tablespoons reduced-fat mayonnaise

6 ounces multigrain French bread, halved lengthwise, then cut in half crosswise (making 4 pieces)

1 medium tomato, halved, seeded, and finely chopped

4 medium apples, sliced

1. Preheat broiler. Combine the ham, onion, cheese, and mayonnaise, stir until well blended.

2. Place the bread on a baking sheet, cut side down. Lightly toast the bread under broiler, about 1 minute on each side.

3. Spread equal amounts of the ham mixture evenly over each bread slice, broil 3 minutes or until beginning to lightly brown. Remove, sprinkle with tomatoes. Serve with equal amounts apple slices for each melt.

Exchanges/Choices

1 1/2 Starch

1 1/2 Fruit

1 Med-Fat Meat

1/2 Fat

Calories	305
Calories from Fat	80
Total Fat	9.0 g
Saturated Fat	2.8 g
Trans Fat	0.0 g
Cholesterol	20 mg
Sodium	600 mg
Total Carbohydrate	48 g
Dietary Fiber	6 g
Sugars	20 g
Protein	11 g

BLT WITH ROSEMARY AIOLI

Serves: 4 • Serving Size: 1 sandwich

Exchanges/Choices

1 Starch
1 Vegetable
1 High-Fat Meat

Calories	230
Calories from Fat	90
Total Fat	10.0 g
Saturated Fat	2.3 g
Trans Fat	0.0 g
Cholesterol	20 mg
Sodium	675 mg
Total Carbohydrate	25 g
Dietary Fiber	10 g
Sugars	5 g
Protein	10 g

8 slices center-cut reduced-sodium turkey bacon
8 low-calorie high-fiber multigrain or whole-wheat sandwich bread
1/4 cup reduced-fat mayonnaise
3/4 teaspoon chopped fresh rosemary, or 1/4 teaspoon dried rosemary, crumbled
1 medium garlic clove, minced
1/2 cup thinly sliced red onion
4 cups loosely packed spring greens
8 (about 8 ounces total) tomato slices

1. Place a large nonstick skillet over medium-high heat until hot, add the bacon until crisp and remove. Blot with paper towels and break each slice in half.

2. Meanwhile, lightly toast the bread slices and set aside. Combine the mayonnaise, rosemary, and garlic in a small bowl.

3. To assemble, spread equal amounts of the mayonnaise mixture (1 tablespoon) on each of four bread slices, top with equal amounts of onion, greens, tomato, and bacon slices. Top with remaining bread slices.

HOT ROAST BEEF SANDWICHES

Serves: 4 • Serving Size: 2 bread slices, 3 ounces cooked beef, and about 2 tablespoons sauce

1 pound boneless sirloin steak

2 teaspoons instant coffee granules

1/4 teaspoon black pepper

1/2 cup water

1/4 cup dry red wine

2 teaspoons balsamic vinegar

2 teaspoons from a 1-ounce package au jus gravy mix (such as McCormick)

1 teaspoon sugar

1/8 to 1/4 teaspoon dried red pepper flakes

6 ounces whole-wheat Italian bread, cut into 8 slices, warmed

2 tablespoons stone-ground or regular Dijon mustard

2 tablespoons chopped parsley (optional)

Exchanges/Choices

1 1/2 Starch

3 Lean Meat

Calories	275
Calories from Fat	55
Total Fat	6.0 g
Saturated Fat	2.0 g
Trans Fat	0.1 g
Cholesterol	40 mg
Sodium	720 mg
Total Carbohydrate	23 g
Dietary Fiber	3 g
Sugars	5 g
Protein	28 g

1. Sprinkle both sides of the beef with the coffee granules and the pepper, pressing down with fingertips to adhere. Place a large nonstick skillet over medium-high heat until hot. Coat skillet with cooking spray and cook beef 4 minutes on each side. Place on cutting board and let stand 3 minutes before thinly slicing.

2. Meanwhile, stir together the water, wine, vinegar, gravy mix, sugar, and pepper flakes in a small bowl and set aside.

3. Add the wine mixture to the skillet and bring to a boil, scraping bottom and boiling 3 minutes or until reduced to a scant 1/2 cup. Remove from heat and stir in the oil. Add any accumulated juices from the beef (on the cutting board).

4. Place two bread slices on each of four dinner plates, spread each bread slice with equal amounts of the mustard (about 1/2 teaspoon), arrange equal amounts of the beef on top of bread slices, spoon the sauce over all, and sprinkle with the parsley if desired.

HOT AND SLOPPY BUNS

Serves: 4 • Serving Size: about 1/2 cup

12	ounces extra-lean ground beef
1	cup diced onion
1	teaspoon sugar or pourable sugar substitute
1	teaspoon chili powder
1/2	teaspoon ground cumin
1/4	cup ketchup
1/4	cup water
1	teaspoon Worcestershire sauce
1	teaspoon cider vinegar
4	whole-wheat hamburger buns

1. Place a large nonstick skillet over medium-high heat until hot. Coat skillet with cooking spray, add the beef, and cook 2 minutes. Add the onion and cook 5 minutes or until translucent, stirring frequently.

2. Meanwhile, combine the remaining ingredients, except hamburger buns, in a small bowl. Stir until well blended and set aside.

3. Add the ketchup mixture to the ground beef, stir, and cook 1 minute to heat thoroughly.

4. Spoon the beef over the open-face buns. Serve with knives and forks, if desired.

Exchanges/Choices

2 Starch
2 Lean Meat

Calories	260	
Calories from Fat	55	
Total Fat	6.0	g
Saturated Fat	1.9	g
Trans Fat	0.2	g
Cholesterol	45	mg
Sodium	460	mg
Total Carbohydrate	31	g
Dietary Fiber	4	g
Sugars	10	g
Protein	23	g

Cook's Note
Make a future meal even quicker by doubling the batch and freezing for later use.

STUFFED GREEK PITAS WITH FETA

Serves: 4 • Serving Size: 2 halves

Exchanges/Choices

2 1/2 Starch
1 Vegetable
1 Lean Meat
1 Fat

Calories	300	
Calories from Fat	70	
Total Fat	8.0	g
Saturated Fat	2.4	g
Trans Fat	0.0	g
Cholesterol	35	mg
Sodium	885	mg
Total Carbohydrate	43	g
Dietary Fiber	7	g
Sugars	4	g
Protein	19	g

1/4 cup light ranch dressing
1 teaspoon dried oregano leaves, crumbled
1 medium garlic clove, minced
4 cups chopped romaine
1 cup precooked diced chicken breast meat
1 cup diced tomatoes
4 whole-wheat or white pitas, cut in half (warmed, if desired)
1/2 cup reduced-fat crumbled feta

1. Combine the salad dressing, oregano, and garlic in a small bowl and set aside. Combine the romaine, chicken, tomatoes in a large bowl, add the dressing mixture, and toss gently, yet thoroughly, until well coated.

2. Fill each pita half with equal amounts of the salad mixture and sprinkle feta evenly over all.

CHICKEN AND PEANUT LETTUCE WRAPS

Serves: 4 • Serving Size: 3 wraps

Sauce

2	tablespoons pourable sugar substitute
2	tablespoons lime juice
1 1/2	tablespoons light soy sauce
1/8	teaspoon dried red pepper flakes

Wraps

3	cups coleslaw mix
1	cup chopped cooked chicken breast meat
1/2	cup chopped green onions
1/2	cup chopped fresh cilantro
1/4	cup (1 oz) unsalted peanuts, preferably toasted
12	romaine or large Boston lettuce leaves

1. Combine the sauce ingredients in a small bowl, stir until well blended, and set aside. Combine the filling ingredients in a medium bowl, toss gently, yet thoroughly, to blend.

2. To assemble, spoon 1/3 cup of the filling into each of the lettuce leaves and then spoon 1 teaspoon of the sauce over each filled lettuce leaf. Roll up.

Exchanges/Choices

1 Vegetable
2 Lean Meat
1/2 Fat

Calories	145	
Calories from Fat	55	
Total Fat	6.0	g
Saturated Fat	1.0	g
Trans Fat	0.0	g
Cholesterol	30	mg
Sodium	260	mg
Total Carbohydrate	9	g
Dietary Fiber	3	g
Sugars	3	g
Protein	14	g

THOUSAND ISLAND TURKEY AND MIXED GREEN SALAD

Serves: 4 • Serving Size: about 2 cups salad and 1/4 cup dressing

Exchanges/Choices

1/2 Carbohydrate
1 Vegetable
1 Med-Fat Meat
1 Fat

Calories	190
Calories from Fat	90
Total Fat	10.0 g
Saturated Fat	2.4 g
Trans Fat	0.0 g
Cholesterol	30 mg
Sodium	395 mg
Total Carbohydrate	13 g
Dietary Fiber	2 g
Sugars	9 g
Protein	13 g

Dressing

2/3 cup fat-free or low-fat buttermilk
1/3 cup reduced-fat mayonnaise
2 to 3 tablespoons ketchup
2 teaspoons sugar
1 1/2 teaspoons cider vinegar
1/2 teaspoon Worcestershire sauce (optional)
Dash cayenne

Salad

6 cups mixed greens
1/2 cup thinly sliced red onion
4 ounces thinly sliced oven-roasted turkey, chopped
1 medium tomato, chopped
1/4 cup shredded reduced-fat sharp cheddar cheese

1. Whisk together the dressing ingredients in a small bowl.

2. Place equal amounts of the mixed greens on each of four dinner plates. Spoon 1/4 cup of the dressing on top of each. Sprinkle evenly with the remaining ingredients in the order listed.

CHICKEN-MANDARIN SALAD WITH GOAT CHEESE

Serves: 4 • Serving Size: 2 cups

6 cups spring greens
1/2 cup thinly sliced red onion
1 11-ounce can mandarin oranges, drained
1/2 cup low-fat sesame ginger dressing
2 cups diced cooked chicken breast meat
1/2 cup reduced-fat feta cheese
1/4 cup hulled sunflower seeds, toasted

1. Arrange spring greens on a serving platter and top with the onions and oranges. Spoon the dressing evenly over all, and sprinkle evenly with the chicken, feta cheese, and sunflower seeds.

Exchanges/Choices

1 Carbohydrate
4 Lean Meat
1/2 Fat

Calories	260	
Calories from Fat	90	
Total Fat	10.0	g
Saturated Fat	2.4	g
Trans Fat	0.0	g
Cholesterol	65	mg
Sodium	660	mg
Total Carbohydrate	15	g
Dietary Fiber	3	g
Sugars	9	g
Protein	28	g

Cook's Note

For a variation, substitute 1 cup quartered strawberries for the mandarin oranges.

SHRIMP ON GREENS WITH CREAMY AVOCADO-BUTTERMILK DRESSING

Serves: 4 • Serving Size: about 2 cups salad and 1/4 cup dressing

Exchanges/Choices

1 Vegetable
1 Lean Meat
1 Fat

Calories	125
Calories from Fat	65
Total Fat	7.0 g
Saturated Fat	1.1 g
Trans Fat	0.0 g
Cholesterol	70 mg
Sodium	255 mg
Total Carbohydrate	6 g
Dietary Fiber	2 g
Sugars	3 g
Protein	10 g

Dressing

- 1 ripe medium avocado, peeled and pitted
- 1 cup fat-free or low-fat buttermilk
- 2 medium garlic cloves, peeled
- 2 tablespoons lime juice
- 2 tablespoons extra virgin olive oil
- 1/2 of a 1-ounce packet dried ranch dressing mix

Salad

- 4 cups mixed greens
- 1 medium tomato, chopped
- 1/2 medium green bell pepper, chopped
- 2 cups cooked shrimp

1. Place all dressing ingredients in a blender, secure lid, and puree until smooth.

2. Arrange equal amounts of the lettuce, tomato, and bell pepper on each of four dinner plates. Spoon 1/4 cup of the dressing over each. Top with equal amounts of the shrimp.

Cook's Note
Cover and refrigerate remaining dressing for a later use.

GREAT BIG SALAD

Serves: 6 • Serving Size: 2 cups

2 ounces French bread, cut in 1/2-inch cubes
1/2 cup fat-free Italian salad dressing
1 tablespoon Dijon mustard
1 1/2 tablespoons dried basil leaves
1 10-ounce bag chopped romaine lettuce
1 medium red bell pepper, thinly sliced
1/2 cup thinly sliced red onion
9 ounces frozen diced cooked chicken, thawed
1 cup reduced-fat feta cheese seasoned with basil and sun-dried tomatoes, crumbled

1. Preheat oven to 350°F.

2. Place bread cubes on baking sheet and bake 12 minutes or until golden. Remove from heat and let cool completely.

3. Meanwhile, in a small bowl, whisk together dressing, mustard, and basil, and set aside.

4. In a large salad bowl, combine romaine, bell pepper, onion, and chicken. Add dressing and toss gently, yet thoroughly, to coat. Add croutons, toss, and top with feta.

Exchanges/Choices

1/2 Starch
1 Vegetable
2 Lean Meat

Calories	155
Calories from Fat	40
Total Fat	4.5 g
Saturated Fat	2.3 g
Trans Fat	0.0 g
Cholesterol	40 mg
Sodium	785 mg
Total Carbohydrate	13 g
Dietary Fiber	3 g
Sugars	5 g
Protein	16 g

SHREDDED CHIPOTLE TACO SALAD

Serves: 6 • Serving Size: 1/6 recipe

Exchanges/Choices

1 Starch

1 Lean Meat

Calories	135
Calories from Fat	30
Total Fat	3.5 g
Saturated Fat	1.9 g
Trans Fat	0.0 g
Cholesterol	10 mg
Sodium	325 mg
Total Carbohydrate	18 g
Dietary Fiber	3 g
Sugars	2 g
Protein	7 g

4 ounces shredded lettuce

3/4 cup canned black beans, rinsed and drained

2/3 cup chipotle salsa

6 tablespoons fat-free sour cream

3/4 cup shredded reduced-fat sharp cheddar cheese

2 ounces baked tortilla chips, crumbled

1. In a 9-inch glass pie pan, layer ingredients in order, starting with lettuce and ending with chips.

RETRO PASTA SALAD WITH HAM

Serves: 4 • Serving Size: 1 1/2 cups

6	ounces uncooked whole-grain penne pasta
2/3	cup extra-lean ham, chopped
1	cup finely chopped green bell pepper
3/4	cup thinly sliced celery
1/4	cup finely chopped red or yellow onion
3	tablespoons sweet pickle relish
1/3	cup reduced-fat mayonnaise

1. Cook pasta according to package directions, omitting any salt or fats.

2. Meanwhile, in a medium mixing bowl, combine remaining ingredients. Mix well and set aside.

3. Drain cooked pasta in colander and run under cold water until completely cooled. Shake off excess liquid.

4. Add pasta to ham mixture and mix gently, yet thoroughly.

Exchanges/Choices

2 1/2 Starch
1 Vegetable
1 Lean Meat
1/2 Fat

Calories	290	
Calories from Fat	70	
Total Fat	8.0	g
Saturated Fat	1.4	g
Trans Fat	0.0	g
Cholesterol	20	mg
Sodium	640	mg
Total Carbohydrate	44	g
Dietary Fiber	6	g
Sugars	9	g
Protein	12	g

TOMATO-MOZZARELLA PENNE SALAD WITH CAPERS

Serves: 5 • Serving Size: 1 1/2 cups

Exchanges/Choices

2 Starch
1 Vegetable
1 Med-Fat Meat
1/2 Fat

Calories	280	
Calories from Fat	80	
Total Fat	9.0	g
Saturated Fat	2.4	g
Trans Fat	0.0	g
Cholesterol	10	mg
Sodium	420	mg
Total Carbohydrate	40	g
Dietary Fiber	6	g
Sugars	4	g
Protein	12	g

8 ounces uncooked dry whole-grain penne or rotini pasta

2 cups cherry tomatoes (preferably sweet grape variety), halved

4 reduced-fat mozzarella cheese sticks, cut into 1/4-inch slices

1/2 cup chopped parsley leaves

1/3 cup capers, drained

2 tablespoons extra virgin olive oil

2 teaspoons dried basil leaves

1 garlic clove, minced

1/4 teaspoon dried red pepper flakes (optional)

1 medium lemon, halved

1. Cook pasta according to package directions, omitting any salt or fats.

2. Meanwhile, in a large mixing bowl, combine remaining ingredients except lemon. Grate 1/2 teaspoon lemon zest and add to the tomato mixture. Squeeze the juice of the lemon over all and set aside.

3. Drain pasta in a colander and rinse under cold water until completely cooled. Drain completely and add to tomato mixture. Salt to taste, if desired. Toss well and serve.

TUSCAN PASTA AND WHITE BEAN SALAD

Serves: 4 • Serving Size: 1 cup

6 ounces uncooked whole-grain rotini

12 kalamata olives, pitted and coarsely chopped

3 tablespoons capers, drained

2 tablespoons finely chopped parsley

2 tablespoons cider vinegar

2 tablespoons extra virgin olive oil

1 tablespoons dried basil leaves

1 garlic clove, minced

1 15.5-ounce can navy beans

4 romaine lettuce leaves

1. Cook pasta according to package directions, omitting any salt or fats.

2. Meanwhile, in a medium mixing bowl, combine olives, capers, parsley, vinegar, oil, basil, and garlic.

3. Place beans in a colander and drain cooked pasta and water over beans. Run pasta mixture under cool water until completely cooled.

4. Shake off excess liquid and add pasta and beans to olive mixture. Mix gently, yet thoroughly.

5. Place a lettuce leaf on each plate and top each with 1 cup pasta mixture.

Exchanges/Choices

3 Starch
1 Lean Meat
1 Fat

Calories	325
Calories from Fat	80
Total Fat	9.0 g
Saturated Fat	1.3 g
Trans Fat	0.0 g
Cholesterol	0 mg
Sodium	425 mg
Total Carbohydrate	49 g
Dietary Fiber	12 g
Sugars	1 g
Protein	12 g

BLACK BEAN, MOZZARELLA, AND RICE SALAD

Serves: 4 • Serving Size: 1 1/2 cups

Exchanges/Choices

2 Starch
1 Vegetable
1 Med-Fat Meat

Calories	265	
Calories from Fat	70	
Total Fat	8.0	g
Saturated Fat	2.6	g
Trans Fat	0.0	g
Cholesterol	10	mg
Sodium	260	mg
Total Carbohydrate	37	g
Dietary Fiber	8	g
Sugars	5	g
Protein	14	g

1	10-ounce package frozen precooked brown rice
1	15.5-ounce can black beans, rinsed and drained
1	poblano chili pepper, finely chopped
1 1/2	cups sweet grape cherry tomatoes, quartered
4	sticks reduced-fat mozzarella cheese, cut into 1/4-inch slices
1/4	cup chopped cilantro leaves
1/4	cup lime juice
1/4	teaspoon dried red pepper flakes
1	tablespoon extra virgin olive oil

1. Cook rice according to package directions, omitting any salt or fats.

2. Meanwhile, in a large mixing bowl, combine remaining ingredients except oil.

3. To cool rice quickly, place on a baking sheet in a thin layer and let stand 5 minutes. Add rice to bean mixture and mix gently. Add oil and, if desired, salt, and mix gently.

1	cup water

LEMONY COUSCOUS AND FRESH SPINACH SALAD

Serves: 4 • Serving Size: about 3/4 cup couscous and 3 tomato slices

3/4 cup whole-wheat or plain dry couscous

1 ounce pine nuts (preferably toasted)

1/2 15.5-ounce can navy beans, rinsed and drained

1 cup loosely packed baby spinach, coarsely chopped

1 tablespoon extra virgin olive oil

2 teaspoons grated lemon zest

1 tablespoon lemon juice

1 teaspoon dried oregano leaves, crumbled

1 medium garlic clove, minced

3 (12 ounces total) medium tomatoes, cut in four slices each

1. Bring water to a boil in a medium saucepan over high heat. Remove from heat, stir in the couscous, cover, and let stand 5 minutes.

2. Meanwhile, combine the remaining ingredients, except the tomato slices.

3. Place the couscous in a fine mesh sieve and run under cold water until completely cooled, shaking off excess water. Add to the spinach mixture and toss gently yet thoroughly until well blended. Season lightly with salt and pepper, if desired.

4. To serve, arrange three tomato slices on each of four dinner plates and spoon equal amounts of the couscous mixture on top of each serving.

Exchanges/Choices

2 Starch

1 Lean Meat

1 Fat

Calories	240
Calories from Fat	90
Total Fat	10.0 g
Saturated Fat	1.0 g
Trans Fat	0.0 g
Cholesterol	0 mg
Sodium	80 mg
Total Carbohydrate	34 g
Dietary Fiber	7 g
Sugars	3 g
Protein	8 g

TOMATO BASIL SOUP WITH CHICKEN

Serves: 4 • Serving Size: 1 cup soup

Exchanges/Choices

1/2 Starch
2 Vegetable
2 Lean Meat
1/2 Fat

Calories	195	
Calories from Fat	45	
Total Fat	5.0	g
Saturated Fat	1.5	g
Trans Fat	0.0	g
Cholesterol	35	mg
Sodium	725	mg
Total Carbohydrate	18	g
Dietary Fiber	4	g
Sugars	6	g
Protein	18	g

1 14.5-ounce can diced tomatoes with Italian seasonings
1/2 15.5-ounce can no-salt-added navy beans, rinsed and drained
1 14-ounce can reduced-sodium chicken broth
1 teaspoon sugar
1 cup cooked chicken breast meat
2 ounces baby spinach
2 tablespoons chopped fresh basil leaves
2 teaspoons extra virgin olive oil
1/4 cup shredded mozzarella cheese

1. Combine the tomatoes, beans, broth, and sugar in a large saucepan. Bring to a boil over high heat, reduce heat, cover, and simmer 5 minutes.

2. Add the chicken, spinach, and basil, and cook 2 minutes or until spinach is wilted. Remove from heat, and stir in the oil.

3. To serve, top each serving with 1 tablespoon mozzarella.

Cook's Note

If cooked chicken is not available, cut 8 ounces uncooked boneless chicken breast into bite-size pieces, and cook over medium high heat 3 to 4 minutes or until no longer pink in center.

SUPER-FAST ITALIAN TOMATO SOUP

Serves: 4 • Serving Size: 1 cup

1   14.5-ounce can stewed tomatoes
1   (about 4 ounces) small zucchini, thinly sliced
1   14-ounce can reduced-sodium chicken broth
2   teaspoons dried basil leaves
1   cup diced cooked chicken breast meat
1   ounce baby spinach leaves
1/2 cup chopped green onions
1/4 to 1/2 teaspoon dried rosemary leaves
1   tablespoon extra virgin olive oil

1. Combine tomatoes, zucchini, chicken broth, and basil in a large saucepan. Bring to boil, reduce heat, cover, and simmer 8 minutes or until zucchini is just tender.

2. Remove from heat, break up large pieces of tomato with a fork, add the remaining ingredients, cover, and let stand 3 minutes to absorb flavors.

Exchanges/Choices

2 Vegetable
1 Lean Meat
1/2 Fat

Calories	120
Calories from Fat	40
Total Fat	4.5 g
Saturated Fat	0.9 g
Trans Fat	0.0 g
Cholesterol	25 mg
Sodium	620 mg
Total Carbohydrate	10 g
Dietary Fiber	2 g
Sugars	5 g
Protein	11 g

CREAMY HAM AND POTATO-OREGANO SOUP

Serves: 4 • Serving Size: 1 cup

Exchanges/Choices

1 Carbohydrate
1 Lean Meat
1/2 Fat

Calories	135	
Calories from Fat	30	
Total Fat	3.5	g
Saturated Fat	1.1	g
Trans Fat	0.0	g
Cholesterol	15	mg
Sodium	665	mg
Total Carbohydrate	18	g
Dietary Fiber	2	g
Sugars	7	g
Protein	9	g

1/2 cup 96% fat-free diced ham
1 cup frozen hash browns, cubed variety (with peppers and onions or plain)
1/2 teaspoon dried oregano leaves
1 1/2 cups 1% milk
1 10.75-ounce can 98% fat-free cream of mushroom soup
1/2 cup chopped green onions

1. Place a large saucepan over medium-high heat until hot. Coat saucepan with cooking spray, add ham, and cook 2 minutes or until beginning to lightly brown on edges, stirring frequently. Remove from saucepan and set aside on separate plate.

2. Coat pan with cooking spray, add the potatoes, oregano, and 1/2 cup of the milk. Bring just to a boil over high heat, reduce heat, cover, and simmer 5 minutes.

3. Add the remaining milk, ham, soup, and onions and cook over medium heat 3 minutes or until heated thoroughly.

HAM AND NAVY BEAN SOUP WITH CARROTS

Serves: 4 • Serving Size: 1 cup

2 cups 96% fat-free diced ham

2 14-ounce cans reduced-sodium chicken broth

1/2 15.5-ounce can no-salt-added navy beans, rinsed and drained

1 cup chopped onion

1/2 cup matchstick carrots

1 teaspoon dried thyme leaves

2 teaspoons extra virgin olive oil

1. Place a large saucepan over medium-high heat until hot. Coat saucepan with cooking spray, add ham, coat ham with cooking spray, and cook 2 minutes or until beginning to lightly brown on edges, stirring frequently.

2. Add remaining ingredients, except the oil. Bring to a boil over high heat, reduce heat, cover, and simmer 8 minutes or until onions are just tender.

3. Remove from heat, stir in the oil.

Exchanges/Choices

1/2 Starch
1 Vegetable
2 Lean Meat

Calories	160
Calories from Fat	35
Total Fat	4.0 g
Saturated Fat	0.7 g
Trans Fat	0.0 g
Cholesterol	25 mg
Sodium	1025 mg
Total Carbohydrate	17 g
Dietary Fiber	4 g
Sugars	5 g
Protein	14 g

GRAB AND GO TACO CHILI

Serves: 5 • Serving Size: 1 cup

Exchanges/Choices

1 Starch
1 Vegetable
3 Lean Meat

Calories	215	
Calories from Fat	30	
Total Fat	3.5	g
Saturated Fat	1.3	g
Trans Fat	0.2	g
Cholesterol	35	mg
Sodium	700	mg
Total Carbohydrate	27	g
Dietary Fiber	6	g
Sugars	8	g
Protein	21	g

12 ounces extra-lean ground beef
1 15.5-ounce can dark kidney beans
8 ounces frozen chopped green peppers
1 14.5-ounce can no-added-salt stewed tomatoes
1 1.25-ounce packet mild taco seasoning mix
1 teaspoon sugar

1. Place a medium saucepan over medium-high heat until hot. Coat with cooking spray, add beef, and brown 4 minutes, stirring occasionally.

2. Place beans and peppers in a colander and run under cold water to rinse beans. Shake off excess liquid and add to beef. Add remaining ingredients, bring a boil, reduce heat, cover tightly, and simmer 10 minutes.

QUICK-SIMMER CHILI SOUP

Serves: 4 • Serving Size: 1 cup

6 ounces reduced-fat breakfast sausage, such as Jimmy Dean

1 16-ounce can dark kidney beans, rinsed and drained

1 14.5-ounce can stewed diced tomatoes with Mexican seasonings

1 cup finely chopped green bell pepper

1 cup water

1 1/2 teaspoons sugar or pourable sugar substitute

1 teaspoon ground cumin

1. Place a large saucepan over medium heat until hot. Coat saucepan with cooking spray, add sausage, and cook 2 minutes or until beginning to lightly brown on edges, stirring constantly.

2. Add remaining ingredients, except 1/4 teaspoon of the cumin. Bring to boil over high heat, reduce heat, cover, and simmer 8 minutes. Break up large pieces of tomato with fork. Remove from heat, stir in remaining 1/4 teaspoon cumin.

Exchanges/Choices

1 Starch
2 Vegetable
1 Med-Fat Meat
1/2 Fat

Calories	225
Calories from Fat	65
Total Fat	7.0 g
Saturated Fat	2.2 g
Trans Fat	0.1 g
Cholesterol	20 mg
Sodium	670 mg
Total Carbohydrate	29 g
Dietary Fiber	7 g
Sugars	8 g
Protein	14 g

Cook's Note

For an even faster recipe, use pre-chopped or frozen and thawed green bell pepper.

APPETIZERS & SNACKS

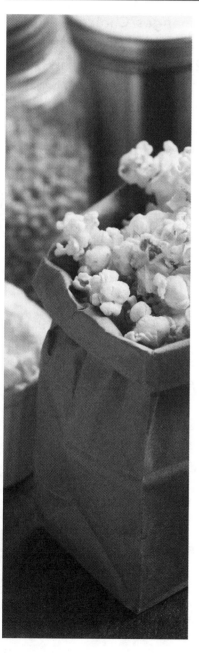

PIZZA MUSHROOMS

Serves: 4 • Serving Size: 4 mushrooms

16 large whole mushrooms, stems removed
3 tablespoons bottled pizza sauce
1/4 cup grated reduced-fat mozzarella cheese

1. Heat oven to 475°F.

2. Arrange mushrooms stem-side up on a nonstick baking sheet and spray mushrooms with cooking spray. Spoon about 1/2 teaspoon of the pizza sauce in the center of each mushroom. Sprinkle mozzarella evenly over mushrooms, about a scant teaspoon per mushroom.

3. Bake 5 minutes or until mushrooms are tender and cheese is lightly golden. Remove from oven.

4. If desired, let stand 5 minutes to absorb flavors and cool slightly.

Exchanges/Choices

1 Vegetable
1/2 Fat

Calories	40
Calories from Fat	15
Total Fat	1.5 g
Saturated Fat	0.8 g
Trans Fat	0.0 g
Cholesterol	5 mg
Sodium	95 mg
Total Carbohydrate	4 g
Dietary Fiber	1 g
Sugars	2 g
Protein	4 g

HOT CHEESY CHIPS

Serves: 8 • Serving Size: 2 chips

Exchanges/Choices

1/2 Carbohydrate
1/2 Fat

Calories	55
Calories from Fat	20
Total Fat	2.5 g
Saturated Fat	1.0 g
Trans Fat	0.0 g
Cholesterol	5 mg
Sodium	130 mg
Total Carbohydrate	6 g
Dietary Fiber	1 g
Sugars	1 g
Protein	3 g

16 baked tortilla chips
1/2 cup grated reduced-fat sharp cheddar cheese
1/2 cup finely chopped poblano chili pepper, or green bell pepper
1/3 cup chopped ripe olives
1/3 cup fat-free sour cream
1/3 cup chopped fresh cilantro

1. Heat oven to 400°F.

2. Place chips on baking sheet and top with equal amounts of cheese, peppers, and olives.

3. Bake 4 minutes or until cheese is melted. Top each with 1 teaspoon sour cream and 1 teaspoon cilantro. Serve immediately.

WHITE BEAN AND SWEET RED PEPPER SALSA WITH PITA WEDGES

Serves: 6 • Serving Size: 1/4 cup salsa plus 6 pita wedges

3	6-inch pita breads, each cut in half
1/2	15-ounce can navy beans, rinsed and drained
1	medium red bell pepper, finely chopped
2	tablespoons lemon juice
1	tablespoon extra virgin olive oil
1	tablespoon capers, drained
1 1/2	teaspoons chopped fresh oregano leaves, or 1/2 teaspoon dried oregano leaves
1/2	medium garlic clove, minced

1. Preheat oven to 350°F.

2. Cut each pita half into 6 wedges. Place on a baking sheet and bake 5 minutes or until just beginning to brown lightly. Cool completely.

3. Meanwhile, combine remaining ingredients in a medium mixing bowl and toss gently, yet thoroughly. Serve with pita wedges.

Exchanges/Choices

1 1/2 Starch
1/2 Fat

Calories	145
Calories from Fat	25
Total Fat	3.0 g
Saturated Fat	0.4 g
Trans Fat	0.0 g
Cholesterol	0 mg
Sodium	255 mg
Total Carbohydrate	25 g
Dietary Fiber	4 g
Sugars	2 g
Protein	5 g

PEPPERONI-JALAPENO MELTS

Serves: 4 • Serving Size: 3 melts

Exchanges/Choices

1 Starch
1/2 Fat

Calories	95
Calories from Fat	35
Total Fat	4.0 g
Saturated Fat	1.5 g
Trans Fat	0.0 g
Cholesterol	10 mg
Sodium	150 mg
Total Carbohydrate	12 g
Dietary Fiber	2 g
Sugars	1 g
Protein	4 g

12 low-sodium Triscuit-style crackers
 6 slices turkey pepperoni, halved
 2 jalapeno chili peppers, each cut in 6 slices cross-wise
1/4 cup shredded reduced-fat sharp cheddar cheese

1. Place crackers in a single layer on a microwave-safe plate. Top each cracker with one pepperoni slice and one jalapeno slice. Sprinkle cheese evenly over all.

3. Cook in microwave on HIGH setting 15 seconds or until cheese just begins to melt.

ARTICHOKE AND PARMESAN DIP

Serves: 12 • Serving Size: 2 tablespoons artichoke mixture plus 6 crackers

2 tablespoons extra virgin olive oil

2 medium garlic cloves, minced

1 13.75-ounce can quartered artichoke hearts, drained and finely chopped

1/4 cup finely chopped roasted red pepper

1 teaspoon dried oregano leaves

1/4 cup fat-free sour cream

1/4 cup grated Parmesan cheese

60 low-sodium Triscuit-style crackers

1. Heat the oil in a medium saucepan over medium-high heat. Cook the garlic 10 seconds, stirring constantly.

2. Stir in the artichokes, roasted peppers, and oregano. Reduce the heat to medium-low, stir in the sour cream, and cook 1 minute.

3. Remove from the heat, stir in the parmesan cheese. Serve with the crackers.

Exchanges/Choices

1 Starch
1 Fat

Calories	140
Calories from Fat	65
Total Fat	7.0 g
Saturated Fat	1.4 g
Trans Fat	0.0 g
Cholesterol	0 mg
Sodium	165 mg
Total Carbohydrate	18 g
Dietary Fiber	4 g
Sugars	1 g
Protein	4 g

Cook's Note

If you want a change from crackers, try serving this with red bell pepper strips, cucumber slices, or yellow squash slices.

MINI BBQ-TOPPED POTATO HALVES

Serves: 4 • Serving Size: 4 potato halves

Exchanges/Choices

1 1/2 Starch
1/2 Carbohydrate
1 Lean Meat

Calories	190	
Calories from Fat	20	
Total Fat	2.0	g
Saturated Fat	1.1	g
Trans Fat	0.0	g
Cholesterol	15	mg
Sodium	390	mg
Total Carbohydrate	34	g
Dietary Fiber	2	g
Sugars	11	g
Protein	9	g

8 (1 pound total) new potatoes, scrubbed and pierced with a fork in several areas
1 cup prepared shredded barbeque chicken
1/3 cup fat-free sour cream
1/4 cup finely chopped green onions

1. Place the potatoes on a microwave-safe plate and cook 5 minutes, turn, and cook another 4 to 5 minutes or until tender when pierced with a fork.

2. Meanwhile, place the barbeque chicken in a small saucepan and heat over medium-high heat, about 2 minutes or until thoroughly heated, stirring frequently. Remove from the heat and cover to keep warm.

3. Place potatoes on cutting board, cut in half lengthwise, top with equal amounts of the chicken, and then top with the sour cream and green onions.

TRIPLE-HERBED TOMATOES

Serves: 7 • Serving Size: 4 tomatoes

1 pint (28) cherry tomatoes, rinsed and patted dry

1 tablespoon lemon juice

1 tablespoon extra virgin olive oil

1 tablespoon chopped fresh basil leaves, or 1 1/2 teaspoons dried basil leaves

1 tablespoon chopped fresh oregano leaves, or 1 teaspoon dried oregano leaves

1 1/2 teaspoons chopped fresh tarragon leaves, or 1/2 teaspoon dried tarragon leaves

1/4 teaspoon salt

1/4 teaspoon black pepper

1. Combine all ingredients in a medium bowl and toss until well blended and thoroughly coated.

Exchanges/Choices

1/2 Fat

Calories	25
Calories from Fat	20
Total Fat	2.0 g
Saturated Fat	0.3 g
Trans Fat	0.0 g
Cholesterol	0 mg
Sodium	85 mg
Total Carbohydrate	2 g
Dietary Fiber	1 g
Sugars	1 g
Protein	0 g

ROASTED PEPPER CROSTINI

Serves: 4 • Serving Size: 2 crostini

Exchanges/Choices

1/2 Starch
1/2 Fat

Calories	70
Calories from Fat	25
Total Fat	3.0 g
Saturated Fat	0.4 g
Trans Fat	0.0 g
Cholesterol	0 mg
Sodium	255 mg
Total Carbohydrate	9 g
Dietary Fiber	1 g
Sugars	1 g
Protein	2 g

2 ounces French bread, preferably baguette-style, cut in 1/4-inch slices (or use regular size French bread, cut into 1/2-inch slices, then cut in half slightly on the diagonal to total 8 pieces)

1/3 cup roasted red peppers, chopped

12 green olives stuffed with pimiento, drained

1/2 teaspoon dried basil leaves

1 teaspoon extra virgin olive oil

1 clove garlic, minced

1. Place bread slices on nonstick baking sheet and lightly coat bread with cooking spray. Place the bread slices in the oven and set the oven to 350°F. (Note: The oven does not have to be preheated.) Bake 5 minutes on each side or until slightly firm. Remove from oven and place on cooling rack to cool slightly, about 2 minutes.

2. Meanwhile, combine the remaining ingredients in a small bowl. Top each bread slice with 1 tablespoon of the pepper mixture.

MINI ANTIPASTO SKEWERS

Serves: 4 • Serving Size: 3 skewers

12	wooden picks, such as toothpicks
1/4	medium green bell pepper, cut into 12 pieces
12	small basil leaves
12	grape tomatoes
1	ounce (1 slice) thinly sliced oven-roasted turkey, cut into 12 pieces
2	sticks reduced-fat mozzarella cheese, cut into 6 pieces each
1 1/2	tablespoons lower-fat balsamic salad dressing

1. Thread each wooden pick with a piece of the bell pepper, basil, tomato, turkey, and mozzarella. Place on a serving platter and spoon salad dressing evenly over all.

Exchanges/Choices
1 Med-Fat Meat

Calories	65
Calories from Fat	25
Total Fat	3.0 g
Saturated Fat	1.4 g
Trans Fat	0.0 g
Cholesterol	15 mg
Sodium	205 mg
Total Carbohydrate	3 g
Dietary Fiber	1 g
Sugars	1 g
Protein	7 g

GOAT CHEESE SPREAD WITH PEARS

Serves: 4, Serving Size: 4 crackers

Exchanges/Choices

1/2 Starch

1/2 Fruit

1 Fat

Calories	115
Calories from Fat	25
Total Fat	3.0 g
Saturated Fat	0.9 g
Trans Fat	0.0 g
Cholesterol	0 mg
Sodium	210 mg
Total Carbohydrate	18 g
Dietary Fiber	1 g
Sugars	6 g
Protein	5 g

1   tablespoon pecan pieces

1/4   cup fat-free cream cheese, softened

2   tablespoons reduced-fat soft goat cheese

16   water crackers

1/2   small firm pear, cored and cut into 16 slices

2   teaspoons honey

1. Place a large nonstick skillet over medium-high heat. Cook the pecans 2 minutes or until fragrant and beginning to lightly brown, stirring frequently. Set aside on separate plate to cool and then chop.

2. Stir together the cream cheese and goat cheese in a small bowl. Spread equal amounts on each of the crackers, about 1 teaspoon each. Top each with a pear slice, drizzle evenly with the honey, and sprinkle the pecans on top.

Cook's Note

To soften cheese quickly, place on a microwave-safe plate and cook on high setting for 10 to 15 seconds.

CROSTINI WITH HERBED BALSAMIC OIL

Serves: 8 • Serving Size: 3 crostini

8 ounces baguette-style French bread
2 tablespoons extra virgin olive oil
1 tablespoon balsamic vinegar
1 tablespoon water
1/2 medium garlic clove, minced
2 teaspoons dried basil leaves
3/4 teaspoon dried oregano leaves
1/4 teaspoon dried rosemary leaves

1. Cut bread into slices 1/2 inch wide, making 24 pieces, and place on a cookie sheet. Set oven temperature to 350°F. (Do not preheat.) Place in oven and bake 10 minutes or until slightly firm to the touch. Remove from heat and place on cooling rack to cool quickly.

2. Meanwhile, in a jar, combine remaining ingredients, secure with lid, and shake vigorously.

3. Brush bread slices with herb mixture.

Exchanges/Choices

1 Starch
1 Fat

Calories	115
Calories from Fat	35
Total Fat	4.0 g
Saturated Fat	0.6 g
Trans Fat	0.0 g
Cholesterol	0 mg
Sodium	185 mg
Total Carbohydrate	17 g
Dietary Fiber	1 g
Sugars	1 g
Protein	3 g

MEDITERRANEAN MORSELS

Serves: 10 • Serving Size: 1/2 cup plus 2 breadsticks

Exchanges/Choices

1/2 Starch
1 Vegetable
1/2 Fat

Calories	95
Calories from Fat	35
Total Fat	4.0 g
Saturated Fat	0.5 g
Trans Fat	0.0 g
Cholesterol	0 mg
Sodium	200 mg
Total Carbohydrate	12 g
Dietary Fiber	2 g
Sugars	2 g
Protein	3 g

12 green olives stuffed with pimiento, drained
 1 cup grape tomatoes
 1 14-ounce can cut hearts of palm, drained
 4 ounces small mushrooms, quartered
1/2 cup canned garbanzo beans, rinsed and drained
1 1/2 tablespoons extra virgin olive oil
 1 tablespoon dried basil leaves
20 plain crisp breadsticks (4 inches by 1/2 inch)
 Wooden toothpicks

1. Combine all ingredients, except breadsticks and tooth-picks, in a gallon-size plastic storage bag. Seal and toss to coat completely. Serve immediately for more pro-nounced flavors, or refrigerate 4 hours to allow flavors to blend.

2. To serve, place on a serving platter with breadsticks and wooden toothpicks.

HUMMUS DIP
Serves: 36 • Serving Size: 1 piece

1	15.5-ounce can garbanzo beans, rinsed and drained
2/3	cup plain fat-free yogurt
2	medium garlic cloves, minced
2	tablespoons lime juice
1/2	teaspoon ground cumin
1/4	teaspoon salt
36	pieces Melba toast

1. Combine all ingredients except Melba toast in a blender, secure lid, and blend until smooth. Top each toast piece with 2 teaspoons dip.

Exchanges/Choices
1/2 Starch

Calories	35
Calories from Fat	0
Total Fat	0.0 g
Saturated Fat	0.0 g
Trans Fat	0.0 g
Cholesterol	0 mg
Sodium	75 mg
Total Carbohydrate	6 g
Dietary Fiber	1 g
Sugars	1 g
Protein	1 g

PEANUTTY DIP

Serves: 4 • Serving Size: 2 tablespoons

Exchanges/Choices

1/2 Carbohydrate
1 Vegetable
1 Fat

Calories	135
Calories from Fat	55
Total Fat	6.0 g
Saturated Fat	0.8 g
Trans Fat	0.0 g
Cholesterol	0 mg
Sodium	310 mg
Total Carbohydrate	16 g
Dietary Fiber	3 g
Sugars	10 g
Protein	5 g

3 tablespoons creamy peanut butter
3 tablespoons apricot or orange 100% fruit spread
1 1/2 tablespoons lite soy sauce
2 tablespoons fat-free milk
1/4 teaspoon ground ginger
24 baby carrots, or 2-inch celery sticks, or 1/2-inch thick apple slices

1. In a small mixing bowl, combine all ingredients, except carrots, celery, or apples. Stir until completely blended. Serve with carrots, celery, or apples.

CREAMY MUSTARD DIPPING SAUCE

Serves: 10 • Serving Size: 1 tablespoon

1/2	cup fat-free or low-fat buttermilk
3	tablespoons reduced-fat mayonnaise
1	tablespoon coarse ground mustard, or Dijon mustard
1/4	teaspoon salt
1/8	teaspoon black pepper

1. Place all ingredients in a small mixing bowl and whisk together until smooth. Cover with plastic wrap and refrigerate until needed.

Exchanges/Choices

Free food

Calories	20	
Calories from Fat	15	
Total Fat	1.5	g
Saturated Fat	0.2	g
Trans Fat	0.0	g
Cholesterol	0	mg
Sodium	145	mg
Total Carbohydrate	1	g
Dietary Fiber	0	g
Sugars	1	g
Protein	1	g

MELON WITH CREAMY DIPPING SAUCE

Serves: 4 • Serving Size: 1/4 recipe

Exchanges/Choices

1/2 Fruit
1/2 Carbohydrate
1/2 Fat

Calories	80
Calories from Fat	20
Total Fat	2.0 g
Saturated Fat	1.4 g
Trans Fat	0.0 g
Cholesterol	10 mg
Sodium	30 mg
Total Carbohydrate	15 g
Dietary Fiber	1 g
Sugars	14 g
Protein	2 g

1/3 cup light sour cream
3 tablespoons powdered sugar
1/2 teaspoon vanilla
1/4 teaspoon coconut extract (optional)
1 teaspoon lime juice
2 cups diced honeydew, or cantaloupe melon, or seedless grapes, or strawberries

1. Combine all ingredients except fruit in a small serving bowl.

2. Place bowl in center of serving platter and arrange fruit around bowl to serve.

VEGGIE DIPPERS

Serves: 5 • Serving Size: 1/2 cup cucumbers plus 1/4 cup dip

1	cup fat-free sour cream
1 1/2	tablespoons dried dill weed
1	tablespoon plus 1 teaspoon extra virgin olive oil
2	teaspoons lime juice
1	teaspoon Dijon mustard
1/2	teaspoon salt
1/4	teaspoon Louisiana hot sauce
2 1/2	cups cucumber slices

1. Place all ingredients except cucumber slices in a small mixing bowl and stir until well blended. Serve with cucumber slices.

Exchanges/Choices

1/2 Carbohydrate

1 Fat

Calories	85	
Calories from Fat	35	
Total Fat	4.0	g
Saturated Fat	0.7	g
Trans Fat	0.0	g
Cholesterol	5	mg
Sodium	315	mg
Total Carbohydrate	10	g
Dietary Fiber	1	g
Sugars	3	g
Protein	3	g

PEARS WITH CINNAMON-CREAM DIPPING SAUCE

Serves: 3 • Serving Size: 1/3 recipe

Exchanges/Choices

1 Fruit
1 Carbohydrate

Calories	145
Calories from Fat	0
Total Fat	0.0 g
Saturated Fat	0.2 g
Trans Fat	0.0 g
Cholesterol	5 mg
Sodium	260 mg
Total Carbohydrate	29 g
Dietary Fiber	4 g
Sugars	21 g
Protein	6 g

4 ounces (1/2 cup) fat-free cream cheese
2 tablespoons sugar
3/4 teaspoon ground cinnamon
1/4 cup fat-free half-and-half, or fat-free milk
1/2 teaspoon vanilla
2 medium pears, sliced

1. Combine cream cheese, sugar, and cinnamon in a small mixing bowl. Using an electric mixer on low speed, beat until well blended.

2. Add half-and-half and vanilla and blend until smooth. Serve with pears.

BEYOND A BAGEL

Serves: 4 • Serving Size: 1 bagel half plus 1/4 cup veggies

2 small (2 ounces each) plain bagels, cut in half

2 tablespoons plus 2 teaspoons reduced-fat cream cheese

1 tablespoon chopped fresh oregano leaves, or 1 teaspoon dried oregano leaves

1/2 cup finely chopped tomato

1 tablespoon plus 1 teaspoon capers, drained

1/2 cup celery sticks

3/4 cup baby carrots

1. Lightly toast bagels in toaster. Spread each half with 2 teaspoons cream cheese.

2. Sprinkle each half with equal amounts of oregano, tomato, and capers. Serve with veggies.

Exchanges/Choices

1 Starch
1 Vegetable
1/2 Fat

Calories	115
Calories from Fat	25
Total Fat	3.0 g
Saturated Fat	1.4 g
Trans Fat	0.0 g
Cholesterol	5 mg
Sodium	280 mg
Total Carbohydrate	19 g
Dietary Fiber	2 g
Sugars	4 g
Protein	4 g

PUMPKIN SEED AND CLUSTER SNACK MIX

Serves: 8 • Serving Size: about 1/3 cup per serving

Exchanges/Choices

1 Carbohydrate

1 Fat

Calories	110	
Calories from Fat	35	
Total Fat	4.0	g
Saturated Fat	1.0	g
Trans Fat	0.0	g
Cholesterol	0	mg
Sodium	175	mg
Total Carbohydrate	19	g
Dietary Fiber	5	g
Sugars	6	g
Protein	3	g

1/2 cup salted pumpkin seeds (in shell)

1/4 cup unsalted peanuts

2 cups (about 4 ounces) high-fiber cluster-style cereal

1/4 cup golden raisins, or dried cranberries

2 tablespoons mini chocolate chips

1. Place a large nonstick skillet over medium-high heat until hot. Cook the pumpkin seeds and peanuts 2 to 3 minutes or until beginning to lightly brown, stirring frequently. Set aside on paper towel in a thin layer to cool quickly, about 5 minutes.

2. Combine the pumpkin seed mixture with the remaining ingredients.

MEXICALI DIP WITH CHIPS

Serves: 13 • Serving Size: 6 large chips plus 2 tablespoons dip

8	slices reduced-fat American cheese
1	cup diced fresh tomatoes, patted dry
1	4-ounce can chopped green chilis
1/2	cup finely chopped green onions
	Louisiana hot sauce, to taste
78	baked tortilla chips

1. Place cheese in a medium microwaveable bowl. Cover with plastic wrap and microwave on HIGH setting 60 seconds. Stir and microwave for 30 or more seconds.

2. Add tomatoes, chilis, and onion. Stir, cover with plastic wrap, and microwave 60 seconds longer or until heated through. Stir in hot sauce, if desired. Serve with tortilla chips.

Exchanges/Choices

1/2 Starch
1/2 Fat

Calories	70	
Calories from Fat	20	
Total Fat	2.0	g
Saturated Fat	1.0	g
Trans Fat	0.0	g
Cholesterol	5	mg
Sodium	265	mg
Total Carbohydrate	10	g
Dietary Fiber	1	g
Sugars	2	g
Protein	4	g

CHEESE TORTILLA ROLLERS

Serves: 4 • Serving Size: 1 roller

Exchanges/Choices

1 Starch

1/2 Fat

Calories	90
Calories from Fat	25
Total Fat	3.0 g
Saturated Fat	1.4 g
Trans Fat	0.0 g
Cholesterol	10 mg
Sodium	125 mg
Total Carbohydrate	11 g
Dietary Fiber	2 g
Sugars	0 g
Protein	6 g

4 soft corn tortillas

1 teaspoon ground cumin

1/2 teaspoon dried red pepper flakes

2 sticks reduced-fat mozzarella cheese, halved lengthwise

1. Place tortillas on a work surface. Sprinkle each tortilla evenly with 1/4 teaspoon cumin and 1/8 teaspoon dried pepper flakes. Place a cheese stick half in the center of each tortilla, roll tortilla around cheese, and place seam side down on a microwave-safe plate.

2. Place in microwave and cook on HIGH setting 30 to 45 seconds or until cheese is just beginning to melt.

3. Remove from microwave and let stand 30 seconds to cool slightly for easier handling.

ON-A-BUDGET BROWN BAG POPCORN

Serves: 2 • Serving Size: 2 1/2 cups

1/4 cup popcorn kernels
1 brown paper sandwich bag
30 pumps butter spray
1/8 teaspoon salt

1. Place popcorn in paper bag, fold edges over twice to seal, place in microwave, and cook on popcorn setting.

2. Remove bag from microwave, spray popcorn 10 times with butter spray, seal bag, and shake. Repeat 2 times, add salt, and shake vigorously to coat completely.

Exchanges/Choices

1 Starch
1 Fat

Calories	115
Calories from Fat	40
Total Fat	4.5 g
Saturated Fat	0.6 g
Trans Fat	0.0 g
Cholesterol	0 mg
Sodium	150 mg
Total Carbohydrate	17 g
Dietary Fiber	3 g
Sugars	0 g
Protein	3 g

SPARKLING FRUIT SMOOTHIES

Serve: 4 • Serving Size: 1/4 recipe

Exchanges/Choices

2 Fruit

Calories	130
Calories from Fat	0
Total Fat	0.0 g
Saturated Fat	0.1 g
Trans Fat	0.0 g
Cholesterol	0 mg
Sodium	35 mg
Total Carbohydrate	31 g
Dietary Fiber	2 g
Sugars	26 g
Protein	2 g

3 cups chopped melon or strawberries, cold
1 medium banana, peeled
1/2 cup frozen orange-pineapple concentrate
1 12-ounce can sugar-free ginger ale

1. Combine all ingredients in a blender, secure lid, and blend until smooth.

PEACH FIZZ SMOOTHIE

Serves: 4 • Serving Size: 3/4 cup

1 cup reduced-fat artificially sweetened vanilla ice cream
1 cup frozen unsweetened peach slices
1 12-ounce can diet ginger ale
1 1/2 tablespoons sugar
1 teaspoon vanilla

1. Combine all ingredients in a blender, secure lid, and blend until smooth.

Exchanges/Choices
1 Carbohydrate

Calories	85	
Calories from Fat	20	
Total Fat	2.5	g
Saturated Fat	1.3	g
Trans Fat	0.0	g
Cholesterol	15	mg
Sodium	30	mg
Total Carbohydrate	16	g
Dietary Fiber	3	g
Sugars	10	g
Protein	1	g

MINTED ESPRESSO HOT CHOCOLATE

Serves: 4 • Serving Size: 1/4 recipe

Exchanges/Choices

1/2 Fat-Free Milk

1 1/2 Carbohydrate

Calories	155
Calories from Fat	0
Total Fat	0.0 g
Saturated Fat	0.3 g
Trans Fat	0.0 g
Cholesterol	5 mg
Sodium	100 mg
Total Carbohydrate	30 g
Dietary Fiber	1 g
Sugars	24 g
Protein	7 g

3 cups fat-free milk

6 tablespoons chocolate syrup

1 tablespoon plus 1 teaspoon instant coffee granules

1/2 teaspoon peppermint extract

1/4 cup fat-free whipped topping

1. Place milk, chocolate, and coffee in a medium microwaveable bowl. Cover with plastic wrap and microwave on HIGH setting for 2 minutes.

2. Stir contents to dissolve coffee granules and microwave on HIGH for 2 more minutes.

3. Remove from microwave, stir in extract, and pour into four individual cups. Top each with 1 tablespoon whipped topping.

STRAWBERRY-APRICOT CREAMERS

Serves: 2 • Serving Size: 3/4 cup

2 cups quartered strawberries

1 cup fat-free atrificially sweetened vanilla ice cream

1 tablespoon apricot 100% fruit spread

1/2 cup ice cubes

1. Combine all the ingredients in a blender, secure lid, and puree until smooth. Pour into two glasses, and serve immediately.

Exchanges/Choices

1 Fruit
1 1/2 Carbohydrate

Calories	160
Calories from Fat	0
Total Fat	0.0 g
Saturated Fat	0.0 g
Trans Fat	0.0 g
Cholesterol	0 mg
Sodium	55 mg
Total Carbohydrate	38 g
Dietary Fiber	6 g
Sugars	23 g
Protein	4 g

Cook's Note

You can easily double this recipe to serve four.

SIDE SALADS

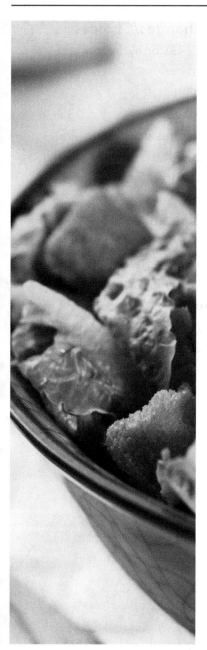

SPRING GREENS WITH RASPBERRY SPICE VINAIGRETTE

Serves: 4 • Serving Size: 1/4 recipe

1 ounce (1/3 cup) sliced almonds

1/4 cup raspberry vinegar

3 tablespoons honey

1/4 teaspoon ground ginger (optional)

1/4 teaspoon ground cinnamon

4 cups prepackaged spring greens

1 cup mandarin oranges, or sliced strawberries, or blueberries

1. Place a large nonstick skillet over medium-high heat. Add almonds and cook 2 minutes or until just beginning to turn golden, stirring frequently. Remove from heat and cool completely.

2. Meanwhile, in a jar, combine vinegar, honey, ginger, cinnamon, and, if desired, salt to taste. Cover with lid and shake vigorously until well blended.

3. Place greens in a salad bowl, add salad dressing, and toss gently. Top with fruit and almonds, and serve immediately.

Exchanges/Choices

1 1/2 Carbohydrate

1 Fat

Calories	135
Calories from Fat	35
Total Fat	4.0 g
Saturated Fat	0.3 g
Trans Fat	0.0 g
Cholesterol	0 mg
Sodium	20 mg
Total Carbohydrate	25 g
Dietary Fiber	2 g
Sugars	22 g
Protein	3 g

SPINACH AND APPLES WITH HONEY MUSTARD DRESSING

Serves: 4 • Serving Size: 1 1/2 cups salad and 2 tablespoons dressing

Exchanges/Choices

1 Carbohydrate
1 Vegetable
1 1/2 Fat

Calories	155	
Calories from Fat	70	
Total Fat	8.0	g
Saturated Fat	0.9	g
Trans Fat	0.0	g
Cholesterol	5	mg
Sodium	155	mg
Total Carbohydrate	21	g
Dietary Fiber	3	g
Sugars	15	g
Protein	3	g

Dressing

3 tablespoons fat-free sour cream
2 tablespoons reduced-fat mayonnaise
2 tablespoons honey
1 tablespoon prepared mustard
1 1/2 teaspoons cider vinegar

Salad

1/4 cup pecan pieces
6 cups baby spinach or spring greens
1/4 cup thinly sliced red onions
1/2 medium green bell pepper, thinly sliced and cut into 2-inch pieces
1 medium red apple (such as Gala), halved, cored, and thinly sliced

1. Whisk together the dressing ingredients in a small bowl.

2. Place a large nonstick skillet over medium-high heat. Add pecans and cook 2 minutes, stirring frequently. Remove from heat and cool completely.

3. Place the spinach leaves on four salad plates and top each with equal amounts of the onions and bell peppers. Spoon the dressing evenly over all. Arrange the apple slices around the salad and top with the pecans.

CAESAR-STYLE SALAD WITH RUSTIC CROUTONS

Serves: 4 • Serving Size: 1 cup

1/2	cup fat-free or low-fat buttermilk
2	tablespoons reduced-fat mayonnaise
1/8	teaspoon garlic powder
1 1/2	tablespoons grated Parmesan cheese
2	ounces French bread or whole wheat bread, torn into 1/2-inch pieces
4	cups prepackaged mixed greens

1. Preheat oven to 350°F.

2. In a small mixing bowl, whisk together buttermilk, mayonnaise, garlic powder, and salt and pepper to taste. Cover with plastic wrap and refrigerate at least 1 hour in order to thicken slightly.

3. Meanwhile, place bread pieces on baking sheet and bake 8 minutes or until slightly firm. Remove from heat and cool slightly.

4. Place mixed greens in a salad bowl, add dressing and cheese, and toss gently, yet thoroughly to coat. Season lightly with salt and pepper, if desired. Add croutons, toss gently, and serve immediately.

Exchanges/Choices

1/2 Starch
1 Vegetable
1/2 Fat

Calories	95
Calories from Fat	30
Total Fat	3.5 g
Saturated Fat	0.8 g
Trans Fat	0.0 g
Cholesterol	5 mg
Sodium	215 mg
Total Carbohydrate	12 g
Dietary Fiber	1 g
Sugars	3 g
Protein	4 g

Cook's Note

Croutons may be made 48 hours in advance, cooled, and stored in an airtight container at room temperature.

ROMAINE WITH CREAMY DILL DRESSING

Serves: 4 • Serving Size: 1 cup lettuce plus 2 tablespoons dressing

Exchanges/Choices

1/2 Carbohydrate

1/2 Fat

Calories	50
Calories from Fat	25
Total Fat	3.0 g
Saturated Fat	0.4 g
Trans Fat	0.0 g
Cholesterol	0 mg
Sodium	175 mg
Total Carbohydrate	5 g
Dietary Fiber	1 g
Sugars	3 g
Protein	2 g

1 0.4-ounce packet buttermilk salad dressing mix

1 cup fat-free or low-fat buttermilk

3 tablespoons extra virgin olive oil

3/4 cup fat-free sour cream

1 tablespoon dried dill weed

4 cups prepackaged Romaine lettuce

1. Combine all ingredients, except lettuce, in a medium mixing bowl and whisk until well blended. Use immediately, or cover with plastic wrap and refrigerate 30 minutes to thicken slightly. (For peak flavors and texture, refrigerate at least 8 hours.)

2. Place mixed greens in a salad bowl, add 1/2 cup of the dressing, and toss gently, yet thoroughly, to coat. Store remaining dressing in refrigerator for later uses.

Cook's Note

You can also use this recipe as a dip for fresh vegetables or tossed with cucumber slices for a quick salad.

ANGEL SLAW WITH ORANGE-GINGER VINAIGRETTE

Serves: 6 • Serving Size: 1/2 cup

3 tablespoons frozen orange-pineapple or orange juice concentrate, thawed

1 tablespoon honey

1 1/2 teaspoons vegetable oil

1 1/2 teaspoons cider vinegar

1/2 teaspoon ground ginger

4 cups finely shredded prepackaged cabbage

1. In a small mixing bowl, combine all ingredients, except cabbage. Using a fork, stir until well blended.

2. To serve, pour over cabbage and toss gently.

Exchanges/Choices

1/2 Fruit

Calories	50
Calories from Fat	10
Total Fat	1.0 g
Saturated Fat	0.1 g
Trans Fat	0.0 g
Cholesterol	0 mg
Sodium	10 mg
Total Carbohydrate	9 g
Dietary Fiber	1 g
Sugars	8 g
Protein	1 g

SWEET AND CREAMY MUSTARD COLESLAW

Serves: 4 • Serving Size: about 3/4 cup

Exchanges/Choices

1 Vegetable

1/2 Fat

Calories	50
Calories from Fat	20
Total Fat	2.5 g
Saturated Fat	0.4 g
Trans Fat	0.0 g
Cholesterol	0 mg
Sodium	115 mg
Total Carbohydrate	7 g
Dietary Fiber	1 g
Sugars	4 g
Protein	0 g

1 tablespoon sugar or sugar substitute

1 tablespoon prepared mustard

2 tablespoons reduced-fat mayonnaise

1 tablespoon water

1 teaspoon celery seed

2 teaspoons cider vinegar

3 cups coleslaw mix

1. Combine all the ingredients, except the coleslaw mix, in a medium bowl. Stir in the coleslaw mix.

BALSAMIC ARTICHOKE AND MUSHROOM SALAD

Serves: 5 • Serving Size: 1 cup

1	14-ounce can quartered artichoke hearts, drained
8	ounces whole mushrooms (preferably small)
16	grape tomatoes
1/2	ounce fresh basil leaves, torn into small pieces, or 1 tablespoon dried basil leaves
3	tablespoons white balsamic vinegar
1	tablespoon extra virgin olive oil

1. Place all ingredients in a gallon zippered plastic bag, seal tightly, and gently toss back and forth to coat completely.

2. Lay on a flat surface and marinate 10 minutes or up to 1 hour, turning occasionally.

Exchanges/Choices

2 Vegetable
1/2 Fat

Calories	75	
Calories from Fat	25	
Total Fat	3.0	g
Saturated Fat	0.4	g
Trans Fat	0.0	g
Cholesterol	0	mg
Sodium	205	mg
Total Carbohydrate	9	g
Dietary Fiber	2	g
Sugars	4	g
Protein	3	g

Cook's Note

To clean mushrooms quickly, lightly wipe with a damp paper towel. Do not soak in water; the mushrooms will absorb excess moisture.

BALSAMIC ASPARAGUS AND HEARTS OF PALM

Serves: 6 • Serving Size: 1/6 recipe

Exchanges/Choices

1 Vegetable
1/2 Fat

Calories	60	
Calories from Fat	20	
Total Fat	2.5	g
Saturated Fat	0.4	g
Trans Fat	0.0	g
Cholesterol	0	mg
Sodium	105	mg
Total Carbohydrate	6	g
Dietary Fiber	2	g
Sugars	4	g
Protein	3	g

1 cup water
18 asparagus spears, trimmed (about 12 ounces)
1 14.5-ounce can hearts of palm, drained
2 tablespoons balsamic vinegar
1 tablespoon extra virgin olive oil
1 teaspoon dried oregano leaves
1 2-ounce jar diced pimiento

1. Bring water to boil in a large nonstick skillet. Add asparagus spears in a single layer, cover tightly, reduce heat, and simmer 2 to 3 minutes or until asparagus is just tender-crisp.

2. Immediately drain into a colander and run under cold water to cool quickly. Drain on paper towels and pat dry.

3. Place asparagus on serving platter and arrange hearts of palm on top.

4. In a small bowl, whisk together the vinegar, oil, and oregano and spoon evenly over all. Sprinkle with the pimiento. Serve immediately for peak flavors and color.

COLD AND CREAMY SWEET CORN SALAD

Serves: 4 • Serving Size: 1/2 cup

2 cups frozen corn kernels
2 tablespoons reduced-fat mayonnaise
1/2 teaspoon sugar
1/8 teaspoon cayenne pepper

1. Combine all ingredients and toss gently. Salt and pepper (preferably coarsely ground), to taste. Serve immediately.

Exchanges/Choices

1 Starch
1/2 Fat

Calories	90
Calories from Fat	25
Total Fat	3.0 g
Saturated Fat	0.4 g
Trans Fat	0.0 g
Cholesterol	0 mg
Sodium	60 mg
Total Carbohydrate	16 g
Dietary Fiber	2 g
Sugars	3 g
Protein	2 g

TOMATOES WITH AVOCADO-PICKLED JALAPENO CUCUMBERS

Serves: 4 • Serving Size: 1/2 cup avocado mixture and 2 tomato slices

Exchanges/Choices

1 Vegetable
1 Fat

Calories	75	
Calories from Fat	55	
Total Fat	6.0	g
Saturated Fat	0.8	g
Trans Fat	0.0	g
Cholesterol	0	mg
Sodium	55	mg
Total Carbohydrate	7	g
Dietary Fiber	4	g
Sugars	2	g
Protein	2	g

1	ripe medium avocado, seeded and chopped
1/2	medium cucumber, peeled and diced
2	tablespoons (about 8 slices) pickled jalapeno slices
2	tablespoons lime juice
2	tablespoons chopped cilantro
2	medium tomatoes, cut in four slices each

1. Combine all ingredients, except the tomatoes, in a medium bowl. Arrange two tomato slices on each of four salad plates. Spoon equal amounts of the avocado mixture on top of the tomato slices. Sprinkle lightly with salt and pepper, if desired.

VEGGIE SALAD ON ROMAINE WITH HAM

Serves: 4 • Serving Size: 1/2 cup plus 1 lettuce leaf

2	tablespoons reduced-fat mayonnaise
2	tablespoons fat-free sour cream
1	tablespoon fat-free milk
1/2	teaspoon sugar
1/4	cup diced lean ham
1/2	cup diced green bell pepper
1/2	cup matchstick carrots
2	tablespoons finely chopped red onion
1/2	cup frozen green peas, thawed
1/4	cup shredded reduced-fat sharp cheddar cheese
1/4	teaspoon coarsely ground black pepper
4	romaine leaves

1. Combine the mayonnaise, sour cream, milk, and sugar in a medium bowl. Stir in the remaining ingredients, except the romaine lettuce. Serve on lettuce leaves.

Exchanges/Choices

1/2 Carbohydrate

1 Fat

Calories	90
Calories from Fat	40
Total Fat	4.5 g
Saturated Fat	1.4 g
Trans Fat	0.0 g
Cholesterol	10 mg
Sodium	240 mg
Total Carbohydrate	9 g
Dietary Fiber	2 g
Sugars	4 g
Protein	5 g

BERRY FRUITY SALAD

Serves: 4 • Serving Size: 1/2 cup

Exchanges/Choices

1 1/2 Fruit

Calories	85
Calories from Fat	0
Total Fat	0.0 g
Saturated Fat	0.1 g
Trans Fat	0.0 g
Cholesterol	0 mg
Sodium	25 mg
Total Carbohydrate	20 g
Dietary Fiber	2 g
Sugars	13 g
Protein	2 g

1/3 cup fat-free sour cream
1 tablespoon pourable sugar substitute
1/2 teaspoon vanilla
1 8-ounce can pineapple tidbits, packed in own juice, drained
1 medium banana, peeled and diced
1 cup whole strawberries, quartered

1. Combine the sour cream, sugar substitute, and vanilla in a medium bowl. Stir in the remaining ingredients.

MANGO-BLUEBERRY SALAD WITH MINT

Serves: 4 • Serving Size: 1/2 cup

1 ripe mango, peeled, pitted, and chopped
1 cup fresh or frozen blueberries, thawed and patted dry
1 tablespoon pourable sugar substitute
1/2 teaspoon grated lime zest
2 tablespoons lime juice
2 tablespoons chopped mint or cilantro

1. Combine all ingredients, except the mint, in a medium bowl. Sprinkle with the mint and toss gently.

Exchanges/Choices
1 Fruit

Calories	65
Calories from Fat	0
Total Fat	0.0 g
Saturated Fat	0.1 g
Trans Fat	0.0 g
Cholesterol	0 mg
Sodium	0 mg
Total Carbohydrate	16 g
Dietary Fiber	2 g
Sugars	13 g
Protein	1 g

APPLE-CHERRY RELISH SALAD

Serves: 4 • Serving Size: 1/2 cup

Exchanges/Choices

1 Fruit
1/2 Fat

Calories	90	
Calories from Fat	20	
Total Fat	2.5	g
Saturated Fat	0.2	g
Trans Fat	0.0	g
Cholesterol	0	mg
Sodium	0	mg
Total Carbohydrate	18	g
Dietary Fiber	2	g
Sugars	14	g
Protein	0	g

1 large (about 2 cups) tart apple, halved, cored and diced
1/4 cup dried cherries, or cranberries
1 teaspoon grated orange zest
1/4 cup orange juice
1/4 to 1/2 teaspoon ground cinnamon
2 teaspoons canola oil

1. Combine all ingredients in a medium bowl. Let stand 10 minutes to absorb flavors.

LEMON-MINTED MELON BOWLS

Serves: 4 • Serving Size: 1 cup

2	cups cubed watermelon
2	cups cubed honeydew melon
1/2	cup red grapes
1/4	cup chopped mint
2	teaspoons grated lemon zest
1/4	cup lemon juice
1/2 to 1	cup diet ginger ale

1. Spoon equal amounts of the watermelon, honeydew, and grapes in each of four dessert bowls. Sprinkle evenly with the mint.

2. Combine the zest and juice in a small bowl and stir until zest is well blended with the juice. Spoon evenly over the fruit and pour the ginger ale over all. Serve immediately for peak flavors and texture. Serve with spoons.

Exchanges/Choices
1 Fruit

Calories	70
Calories from Fat	0
Total Fat	0.0 g
Saturated Fat	0.1 g
Trans Fat	0.0 g
Cholesterol	0 mg
Sodium	25 mg
Total Carbohydrate	18 g
Dietary Fiber	2 g
Sugars	15 g
Protein	1 g

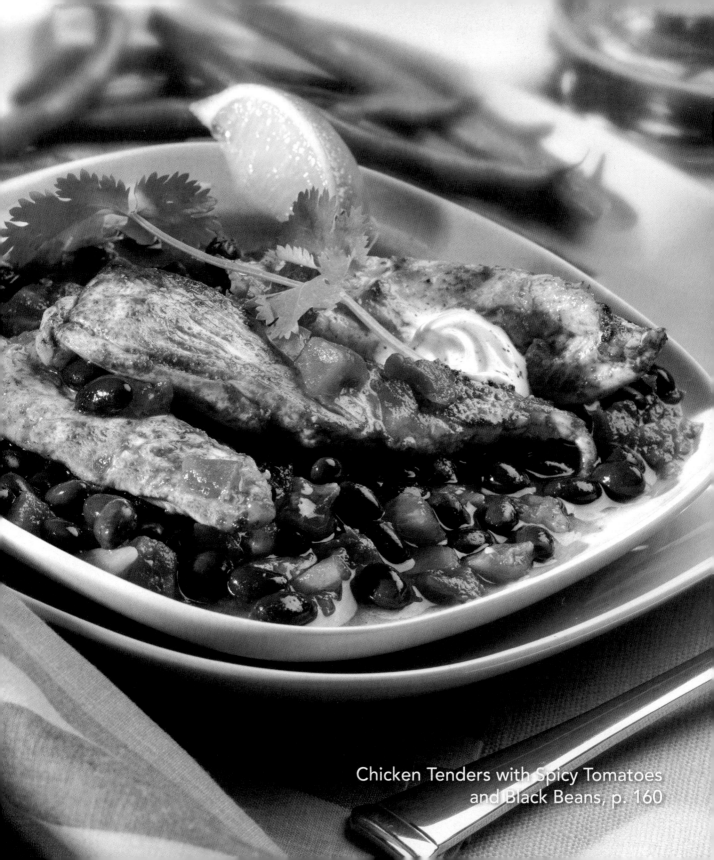

Chicken Tenders with Spicy Tomatoes
and Black Beans, p. 160

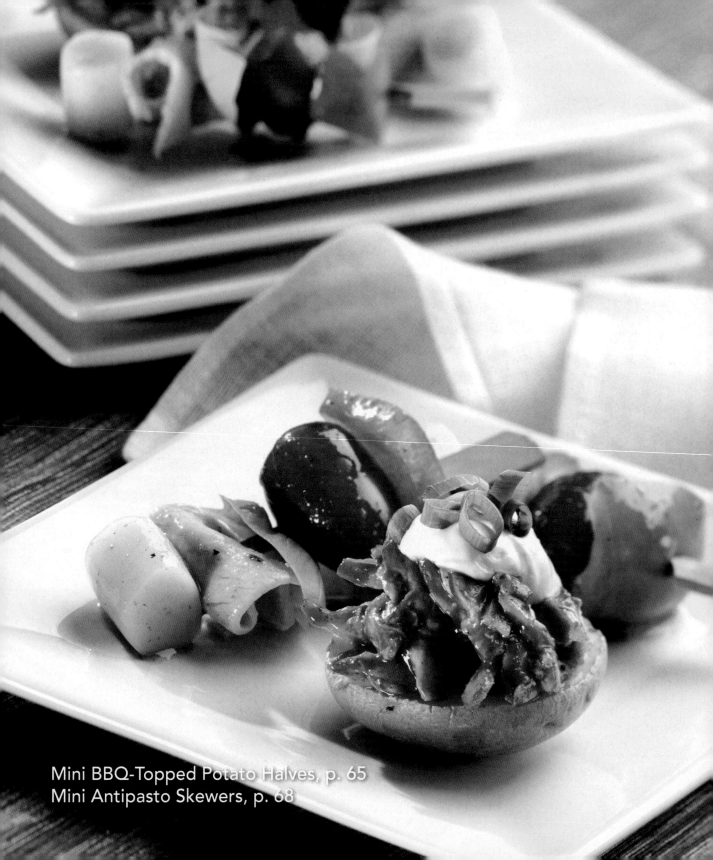

Mini BBQ-Topped Potato Halves, p. 65
Mini Antipasto Skewers, p. 68

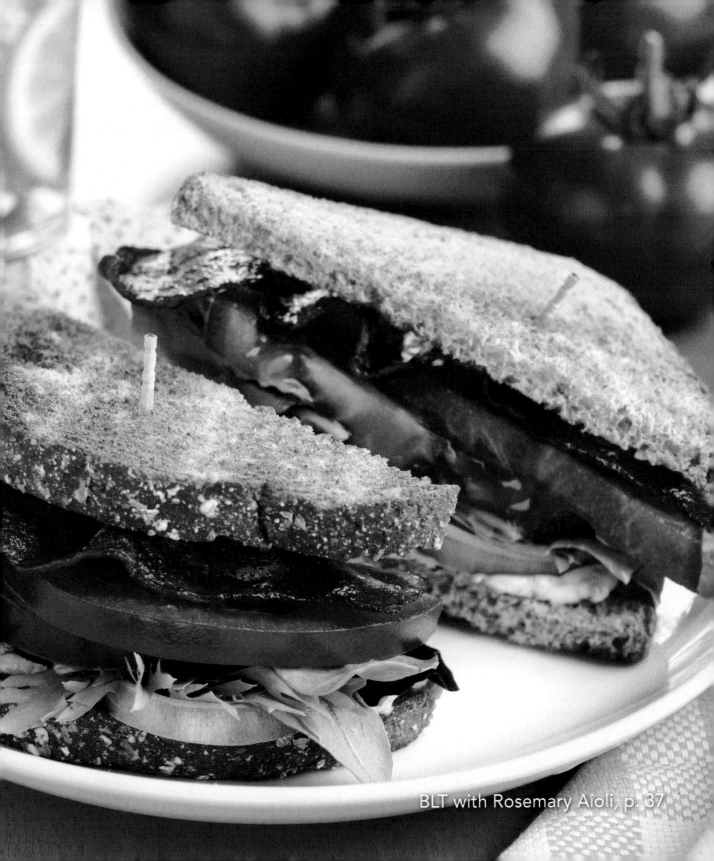

BLT with Rosemary Aïoli, p. 37

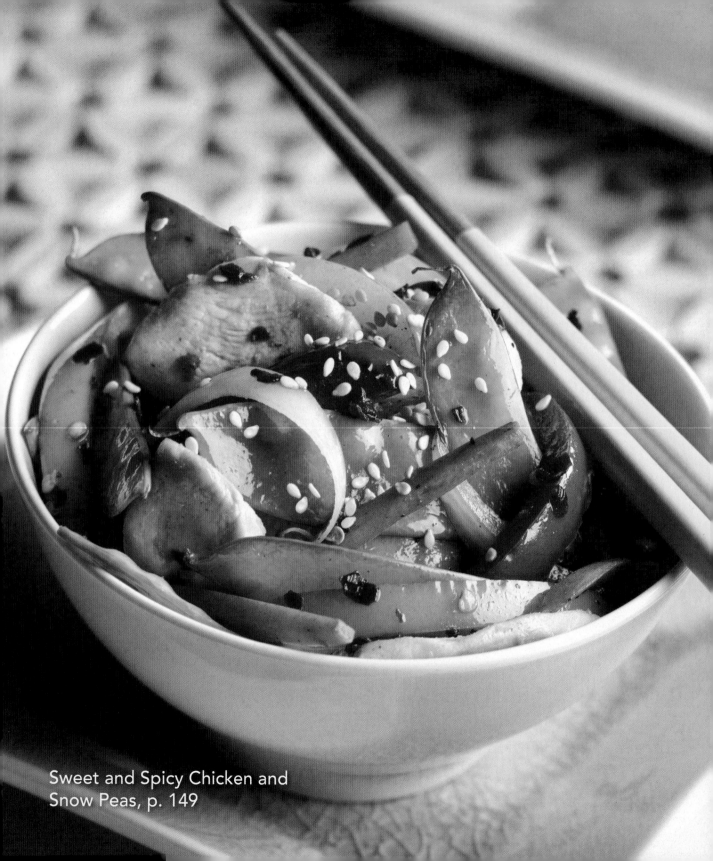

Sweet and Spicy Chicken and
Snow Peas, p. 149

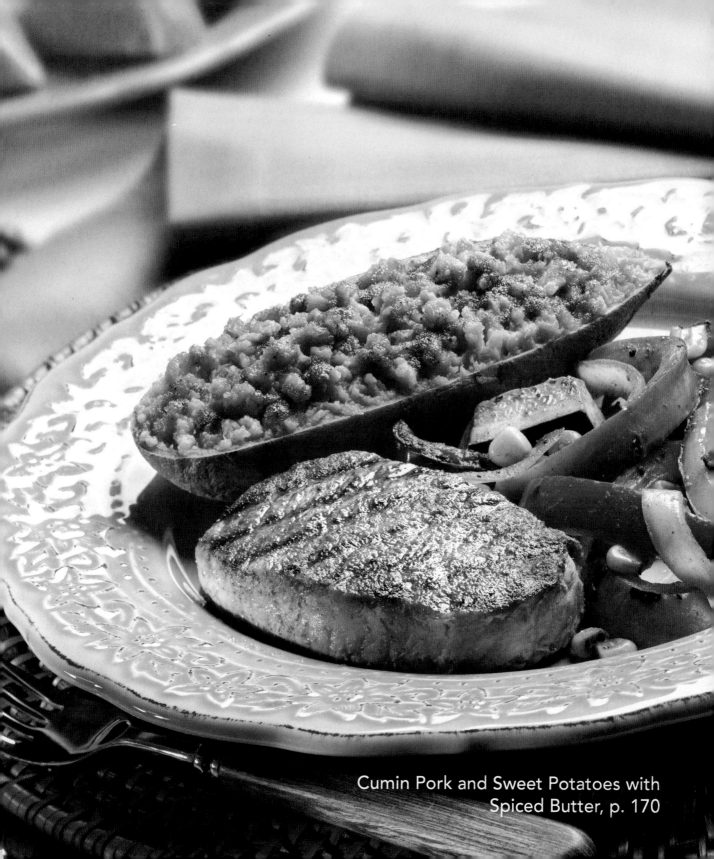

Cumin Pork and Sweet Potatoes with
Spiced Butter, p. 170

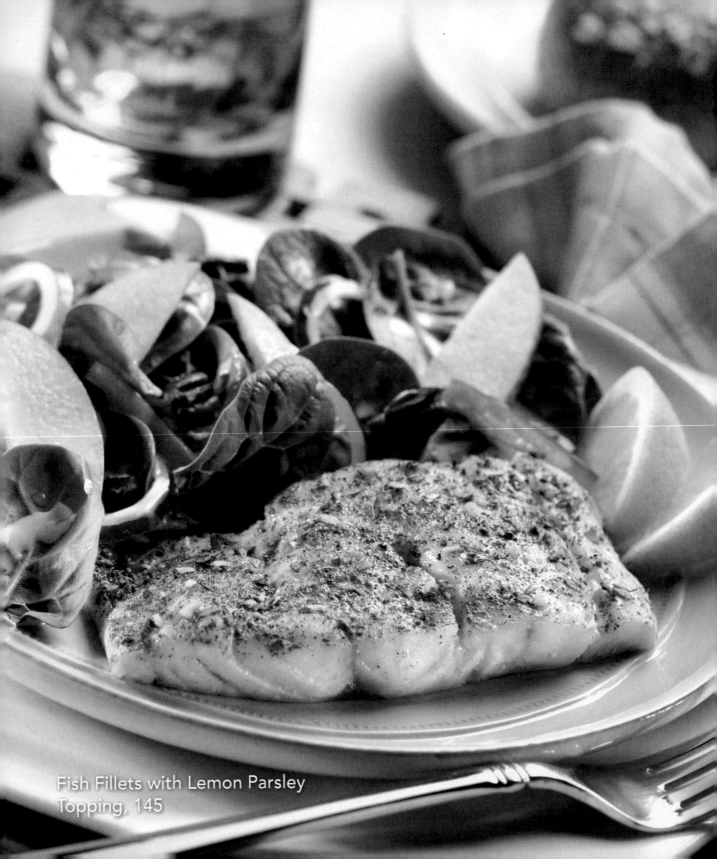

Fish Fillets with Lemon Parsley
Topping, 145

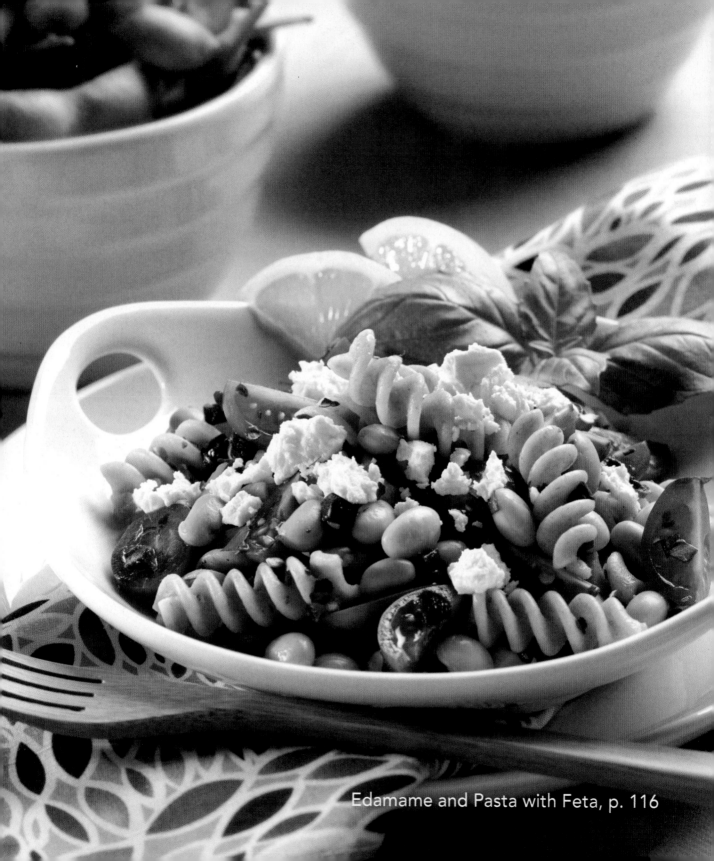

Edamame and Pasta with Feta, p. 116

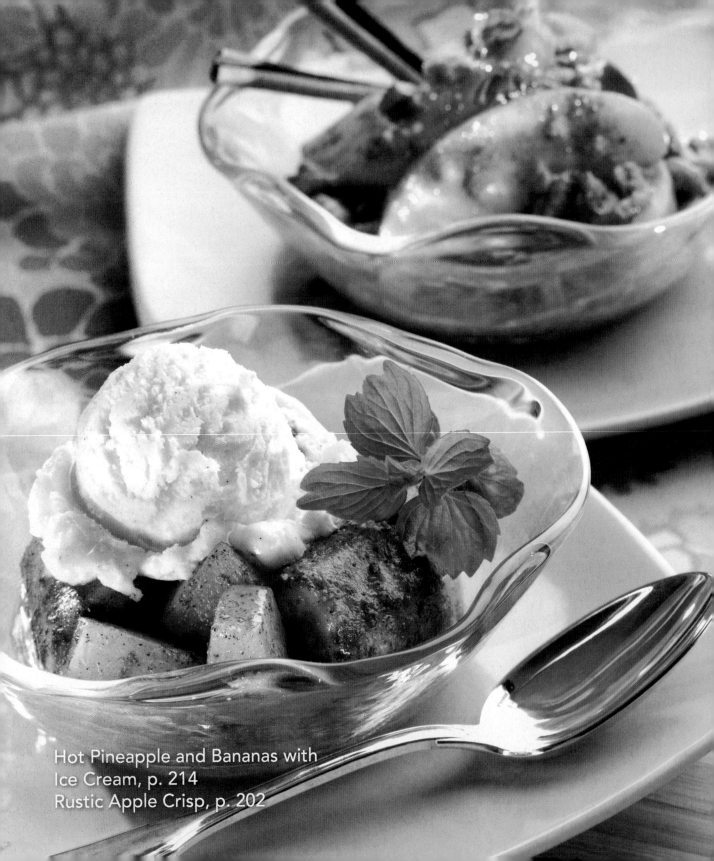

Hot Pineapple and Bananas with
Ice Cream, p. 214
Rustic Apple Crisp, p. 202

COUSCOUS SALAD WITH CAPERS AND OLIVES

Serves: 5 • Serving Size: 1/2 cup

Exchanges/Choices

1 Starch

Calories	80
Calories from Fat	25
Total Fat	3.0 g
Saturated Fat	0.4 g
Trans Fat	0.0 g
Cholesterol	0 mg
Sodium	130 mg
Total Carbohydrate	12 g
Dietary Fiber	1 g
Sugars	0 g
Protein	2 g

3/4 cup water
1/2 cup dried uncooked couscous (preferably whole wheat)
2 tablespoons sliced ripe olives, drained
2 tablespoons capers, rinsed and drained
2 tablespoons lemon juice
2 teaspoons extra virgin olive oil
3/4 teaspoon dried oregano leaves

1. In a small saucepan, bring water to a boil, stir in couscous, cover tightly, and then remove from heat. Let stand about 5 minutes.

2. Fluff couscous with a fork. Cool by placing hot couscous on a baking sheet or sheet of foil in a thin layer, about 5 minutes.

3. Meanwhile, in a medium bowl, combine remaining ingredients.

4. When couscous is completely cooled, combine with dressing and toss gently. Add black pepper to taste, if desired.

BABY SPINACH AND PASTA SALAD

Serves: 7 • Serving Size: 1 cup

3	ounces uncooked whole-grain corkscrew pasta
3	ounces prepackaged baby spinach
2	tablespoons balsamic vinegar
1 1/2	teaspoons dried oregano or basil leaves
1/3	cup feta cheese with basil and sun-dried tomatoes, crumbled
12	pitted kalamata or ripe olives

1. Cook pasta according to package directions, omitting any salt or fats. Drain and rinse under cold water to cool quickly. Shake off excess liquid.

2. Combine pasta, spinach, vinegar, oregano, and 1/4 teaspoon salt, if desired, in a salad bowl. Add the feta and olives and toss gently. Serve immediately for peak flavors.

Exchanges/Choices

1/2 Starch
1 Vegetable
1/2 Fat

Calories	80
Calories from Fat	20
Total Fat	2.5 g
Saturated Fat	1.1 g
Trans Fat	0.0 g
Cholesterol	5 mg
Sodium	115 mg
Total Carbohydrate	11 g
Dietary Fiber	2 g
Sugars	1 g
Protein	3 g

CREAMY PEA AND MACARONI SALAD

Serves: 4 • Serving Size: 1/2 cup

Exchanges/Choices

1 Starch

1/2 Fat

Calories	95	
Calories from Fat	20	
Total Fat	2.5	g
Saturated Fat	0.4	g
Trans Fat	0.0	g
Cholesterol	0	mg
Sodium	85	mg
Total Carbohydrate	16	g
Dietary Fiber	3	g
Sugars	2	g
Protein	4	g

2 ounces uncooked dry whole-grain elbow macaroni

1 cup frozen green peas, partially thawed

2 tablespoons reduced-fat mayonnaise

1/2 teaspoon dried dill weed

1. Cook pasta according to package directions, omitting any salt or fats. Drain and rinse under cold water to cool quickly. Shake off excess liquid.

2. Place pasta in mixing bowl with remaining ingredients, stir to blend thoroughly, and serve immediately. Salt and pepper to taste.

OLIVE OIL AND VINEGAR WARM POTATO SALAD

Serves: 8 • Serving Size: 1/2 cup

4	cups hot water
1	pound red potatoes, diced
2	tablespoons extra virgin olive oil
1	tablespoon cider vinegar
2	teaspoons dried oregano leaves
1	medium garlic clove, minced
1/2	teaspoon salt
1/4	teaspoon black pepper
1/4	cup finely chopped red onion

1. Bring water to boil in a medium saucepan over high heat. Add the potatoes, return to a boil, reduce heat, cover tightly, and simmer 5 minutes or until just tender.

2. Meanwhile, combine the remaining ingredients in a medium bowl.

3. Drain the potatoes in a colander, run under cold water briefly, about 10 seconds, and shake off excess water. Stir the potatoes into the onion mixture. Serve warm or chilled.

Exchanges/Choices

1 Starch
1/2 Fat

Calories	90
Calories from Fat	30
Total Fat	3.5 g
Saturated Fat	0.5 g
Trans Fat	0.0 g
Cholesterol	0 mg
Sodium	150 mg
Total Carbohydrate	14 g
Dietary Fiber	1 g
Sugars	1 g
Protein	1 g

Cook's Note

Placing a lid on the pot will help to bring it to a boil faster.

RED POTATO AND RED ONION SALAD WITH DILL

Serves: 5 • Serving Size: 1/2 cup

Exchanges/Choices

1 Starch

1/2 Fat

Calories	100	
Calories from Fat	20	
Total Fat	2.0	g
Saturated Fat	0.3	g
Trans Fat	0.0	g
Cholesterol	0	mg
Sodium	60	mg
Total Carbohydrate	19	g
Dietary Fiber	2	g
Sugars	2	g
Protein	2	g

2 cups water

12 ounces red potatoes, diced

1/2 cup finely chopped red onion

2 tablespoons fat-free sour cream

2 tablespoons reduced-fat mayonnaise

1 teaspoon dried dill weed

1. Bring water to a boil over high heat in a large saucepan. Add the potatoes, return to a boil, and boil 5 to 6 minutes or until just tender. Drain in colander and immediately run under cold water to cool completely, shaking off excess liquid.

2. Meanwhile, combine the remaining ingredients in a medium bowl. Add the potatoes and toss gently. Season lightly with salt and pepper to taste, if desired.

MEATLESS ENTREES

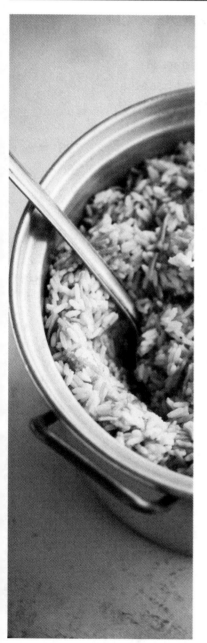

MEDITERRANEAN VEGETABLE STIR-FRY WITH FETA

Serves: 4 • Serving Size: 1/4 recipe

6 ounces uncooked whole-grain rotini pasta

1 tablespoon extra virgin olive oil

1 cup prechopped yellow onion

1 medium green bell pepper, thinly sliced

1 medium zucchini, quartered lengthwise, then cut into 2-inch pieces

1 tablespoon dried basil leaves

1 pint cherry tomatoes (preferably sweet grape variety), quartered

16 pitted kalamata olives, coarsely chopped

3/4 cup reduced-fat feta seasoned with sun-dried tomatoes and basil, crumbled

1. Cook pasta according to package directions, omitting any salt or fats.

2. Meanwhile, place a medium saucepot over medium-high heat until hot. Coat pot with cooking spray and add 1 teaspoon oil.

3. Add onion, bell pepper, zucchini, and basil and cook 5 to 7 minutes or until zucchini is tender crisp and beginning to brown on the edges, stirring frequently.

4. Remove pot from heat and stir in tomatoes, olives, and remaining oil. Cover tightly and let stand 5 minutes to allow flavors to blend.

5. Drain pasta and place in a shallow pasta bowl, top with zucchini mixture, and sprinkle evenly with feta.

Exchanges/Choices

2 Starch
2 Vegetable
1 Med-Fat Meat
1/2 Fat

Calories	295	
Calories from Fat	80	
Total Fat	9.0	g
Saturated Fat	2.7	g
Trans Fat	0.0	g
Cholesterol	5	mg
Sodium	440	mg
Total Carbohydrate	43	g
Dietary Fiber	8	g
Sugars	6	g
Protein	13	g

PIZZA MOUNDS

Serves: 4 • Serving Size: 1/4 recipe

Exchanges/Choices

1 Starch
1 Fruit
1 Med-Fat Meat

Calories	205	
Calories from Fat	45	
Total Fat	5.0	g
Saturated Fat	2.4	g
Trans Fat	0.0	g
Cholesterol	15	mg
Sodium	405	mg
Total Carbohydrate	33	g
Dietary Fiber	6	g
Sugars	11	g
Protein	10	g

2 whole-wheat pita breads
1/2 cup bottled pizza sauce, or spaghetti sauce
4 ounces sliced mushrooms
1 teaspoon dried basil leaves
1 1/2 ounces red onion, thinly sliced
3/4 cup shredded part-skim mozzarella cheese

1. Heat oven to 400°F.

2. Using a serrated knife, cut each pita in half, creating 4 thin rounds like individual pizzas.

3. Top each round with equal amounts of the remaining ingredients in the order listed.

4. Bake 7 minutes or until edges are lightly golden.

SPINACH-ONION FRITTATA

Serves: 6 • Serving Size: 1/6 recipe

1	10-ounce package frozen chopped spinach, thawed and squeezed dry
1/2	cup low-fat small curd cottage cheese
1	cup egg substitute
1	teaspoon dried oregano leaves
1/8	teaspoon cayenne
1	14-ounce can artichoke hearts, drained and coarsely chopped
1	cup diced yellow onion
1	cup shredded reduced-fat sharp cheddar cheese

Exchanges/Choices

2 Vegetable
1 Med-Fat Meat

Calories	140
Calories from Fat	40
Total Fat	4.5 g
Saturated Fat	2.5 g
Trans Fat	0.0 g
Cholesterol	15 mg
Sodium	515 mg
Total Carbohydrate	10 g
Dietary Fiber	3 g
Sugars	3 g
Protein	14 g

Cook's Note

This dish reheats well and makes for excellent leftovers.

1. Preheat broiler.

2. In a medium bowl, combine spinach, cottage cheese, egg substitute, oregano, salt (if desired), and cayenne. Blend well, stir in artichokes, and set aside.

3. Place a large nonstick skillet over medium heat until hot. Coat skillet with cooking spray and cook onion 6 to 8 minutes or until translucent, stirring frequently.

4. Reduce heat to medium low. Add spinach mixture and spread evenly over bottom of skillet. Cover tightly, and cook 15 minutes or until almost set. (The frittata will be very moist at this point because of all the onion. It will set when the cheese is added.)

5. Sprinkle cheese evenly over all and broil 1 to 2 minutes to melt cheese and finish cooking. Remove from broiler and let stand 5 minutes to allow flavors to blend. Cut into 6 wedges to serve.

BLACK BEAN AND GREEN CHILI SKILLET CASSEROLE

Serves: 4 • Serving Size: 1 1/2 cups

1	teaspoon canola oil
1 1/2	cups chopped onion
1	10-ounce package frozen whole-grain brown rice
5	ounces sweet grape cherry tomatoes, quartered
1	15-ounce can black beans, rinsed and drained
1	4-ounce can chopped green chilis
3/4	teaspoon ground cumin
1/4	teaspoon turmeric, optional
1	medium lime, cut in half
1/2	cup shredded reduced-fat sharp cheddar cheese

1. Place a large nonstick skillet over medium-high heat until hot. Add the oil and cook the onions 8 minutes or until richly browned, stirring frequently.

2. Meanwhile, cook the rice in the microwave according to directions on the package. Add the cooked rice, tomatoes, beans, chilies, cumin, and turmeric to the onions in the skillet, stir gently, yet thoroughly to blend. Cook 1 to 2 minutes to heat through.

3. Squeeze half of the lime evenly over all and sprinkle with cheese. Serve with remaining lime half, cut into 4 wedges.

Exchanges/Choices

2 Starch
1 Vegetable
1 Lean Meat
1/2 Fat

Calories	255
Calories from Fat	45
Total Fat	5.0 g
Saturated Fat	2.1 g
Trans Fat	0.0 g
Cholesterol	10 mg
Sodium	245 mg
Total Carbohydrate	40 g
Dietary Fiber	9 g
Sugars	5 g
Protein	12 g

PEASANT-STYLE WHITE BEANS AND RICE

Serves: 4 • Serving Size: 1 cup

Exchanges/Choices

2 Starch
1 Lean Meat
1/2 Fat

Calories	225	
Calories from Fat	70	
Total Fat	8.0	g
Saturated Fat	1.1	g
Trans Fat	0.0	g
Cholesterol	0	mg
Sodium	135	mg
Total Carbohydrate	32	g
Dietary Fiber	8	g
Sugars	0	g
Protein	7	g

1 10-ounce package frozen whole-grain brown rice
1 15.5-ounce can navy beans
3 tablespoons chopped fresh basil leaves, or 1 tablespoon dried basil leaves
2 tablespoons chopped fresh parsley
2 tablespoons extra virgin olive oil
1 lemon, cut into 8 wedges (optional)

1. Cook rice in microwave according to directions on package and set aside.

2. Place the beans in a colander and run under hot tap water until well rinsed and slightly warmed, drain well.

3. Place rice and beans in a shallow bowl, such as a pasta bowl, and top with the basil and parsley. Lightly season with salt and very gently toss. Drizzle oil over all. Do not stir. Serve immediately. May serve with lemon wedges, if desired.

EDAMAME AND PASTA WITH FETA

Serves: 4 • Serving Size: 1 1/2 cups

4	ounces uncooked whole-grain penne or rotini pasta
8	ounces fresh or frozen shelled edamame
1 1/2	cups sweet grape tomatoes, quartered
16	pitted kalamata olives, coarsely chopped
2	tablespoons chopped fresh basil leaves, or 2 teaspoons dried basil leaves
1/2	teaspoon dried rosemary leaves, crumbled (optional)
1	medium garlic clove, minced
1/8	teaspoon dried red pepper flakes (optional)
1	medium lemon, halved, optional
2	ounces crumbled reduced-fat feta

Exchanges/Choices

2 Starch
1 Lean Meat
1 Fat

Calories	235
Calories from Fat	65
Total Fat	7.0 g
Saturated Fat	1.9 g
Trans Fat	0.0 g
Cholesterol	5 mg
Sodium	340 mg
Total Carbohydrate	32 g
Dietary Fiber	7 g
Sugars	4 g
Protein	13 g

1. Cook pasta according to package directions, omitting any salt or fats and adding the edamame during the last 2 minutes of cooking time.

2. In a small bowl, combine tomatoes, olives, basil, rosemary, garlic, and pepper flakes. Toss to blend and set aside.

3. Drain pasta and edamame in a colander, place on serving platter or pasta bowl, squeeze lemon over all, top with feta, and mound the tomato mixture in the center.

COUNTRY SKILLET RICE CASSEROLE

Serves: 4 • Serving Size: 1 cup

Exchanges/Choices

2 1/2 Starch
1 Vegetable
2 Fat

Calories	325
Calories from Fat	110
Total Fat	12.0 g
Saturated Fat	3.3 g
Trans Fat	0.0 g
Cholesterol	20 mg
Sodium	705 mg
Total Carbohydrate	45 g
Dietary Fiber	5 g
Sugars	5 g
Protein	10 g

1 1/2 cups water
3/4 cup uncooked quick-cooking brown rice
2 cups small broccoli florets
1 medium red bell pepper, diced
1 cup frozen corn kernels, thawed
1 10.75-ounce can 98% fat-free cream of mushroom soup
1/3 cup reduced-fat mayonnaise
1/2 teaspoon curry powder
1/2 cup shredded reduced-fat sharp cheddar cheese

1. Bring the water to a boil in a medium nonstick skillet over medium-high heat. Stir in the rice, reduce heat, cover tightly, and simmer 10 minutes, adding the broccoli, bell pepper, and corn during the last 5 minutes of cooking.

2. Meanwhile, combine the soup, mayonnaise, and curry in a small saucepan and place over medium-high heat about 2 minutes or until warm.

3. Spoon the soup mixture over the rice mixture, sprinkle with the cheese and cook, covered, 1 minute to melt cheese slightly.

Cook's Note

To save time, prep the veggies while the rice is cooking during the first 5 minutes. To thaw frozen corn quickly, place in a colander and run under cold water 15 to 20 seconds, making sure to shake off the extra liquid.

SPEED-BAKED STUFFED POTATOES

Serves: 4 • Serving Size: 1 potato and about 1/3 cup mushroom mixture

4 6-ounce red potatoes, scrubbed, and pierced with a fork in several areas
1 teaspoon canola oil
1 cup chopped onion
8 ounces sliced mushrooms
2 medium garlic cloves, minced
1 tablespoon reduced-fat margarine
1/2 cup fat-free sour cream
1/2 cup shredded reduced-fat sharp cheddar cheese

1. Place potatoes in the microwave and cook on HIGH setting 11 minutes or until tender when pierced with a fork.

2. Meanwhile, heat the oil in a large nonstick skillet over medium-high heat. Cook the onions 2 minutes, add the mushrooms, and cook 5 minutes or until beginning to brown, stirring frequently. Stir in the garlic and cook 10 seconds. Remove from the heat and stir in the margarine until melted.

3. Split the potatoes almost in half, fluff with a fork, spoon equal amounts of the sour cream and cheese over each potato, and spoon the mushroom mixture on top. Lightly season with salt and pepper, if desired.

Exchanges/Choices
2 1/2 Starch
1 Vegetable
1 Fat

Calories	265
Calories from Fat	55
Total Fat	6.0 g
Saturated Fat	2.4 g
Trans Fat	0.0 g
Cholesterol	15 mg
Sodium	190 mg
Total Carbohydrate	44 g
Dietary Fiber	4 g
Sugars	5 g
Protein	10 g

MUSHROOM-BASIL TOMATO SAUCE ON PENNE

Serves: 4 • Serving Size: 3/4 cup cooked pasta and about 3/4 cup sauce

Exchanges/Choices

3 Starch

1 Lean Meat

Calories	280
Calories from Fat	55
Total Fat	6.0 g
Saturated Fat	2.4 g
Trans Fat	0.0 g
Cholesterol	10 mg
Sodium	800 mg
Total Carbohydrate	47 g
Dietary Fiber	7 g
Sugars	10 g
Protein	13 g

6	ounces uncooked dry whole-grain penne pasta
4	ounces sliced mushrooms
2	cups bottled spaghetti sauce
1/2	cup chopped roasted red peppers (optional)
1	teaspoon sugar
12	pitted kalamata olives, coarsely chopped
1/4	cup chopped fresh basil leaves, or 1 tablespoon dried basil leaves
1/2	cup shredded part-skim mozzarella cheese
2	tablespoons grated Parmesan cheese

1. Cook pasta according to package directions, omitting any salt or fats.

2. Meanwhile, place a large nonstick skillet over medium-high heat until hot. Coat skillet with cooking spray, add mushrooms, coat those with cooking spray, and cook 5 minutes or until mushrooms are tender, stirring frequently. Stir in the spaghetti sauce, roasted peppers, and sugar, and cover and simmer 5 minutes to absorb flavors.

3. Remove from heat and stir in the olives and basil.

4. Spoon the sauce over the drained pasta and sprinkle evenly with the mozzarella and Parmesan cheeses.

BEEF ENTREES

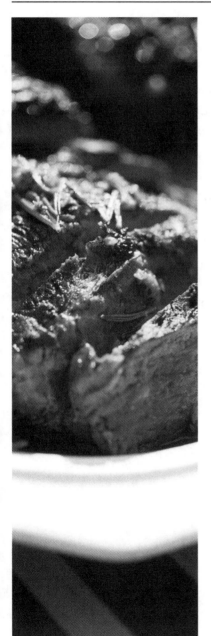

SEARED SIRLOIN WITH SWEET BALSAMIC SAUCE

Serves: 4 • Serving Size: 1/4 recipe

1 pound boneless sirloin steak, about 1-inch thick, trimmed of fat

1/4 cup water

1 tablespoon light soy sauce

1 tablespoon balsamic vinegar

1 tablespoon sugar

1. Place a large nonstick skillet over medium-high heat until hot. Add beef and cook 4 minutes. Turn and cook 4 minutes longer or until beef is done to your liking.

2. Meanwhile, in a small bowl, combine remaining ingredients. Stir to blend and set aside.

3. When beef is done, place on cutting board and let stand. Add sauce mixture to pan residue in skillet. Bring to a boil over medium-high heat and cook 1 to 2 minutes, scraping bottom and sides of skillet.

4. Thinly slice beef and spoon sauce over all.

Exchanges/Choices
3 Lean Meat

Calories	150
Calories from Fat	35
Total Fat	4.0 g
Saturated Fat	1.6 g
Trans Fat	0.1 g
Cholesterol	40 mg
Sodium	190 mg
Total Carbohydrate	4 g
Dietary Fiber	0 g
Sugars	4 g
Protein	23 g

SIRLOIN STEAKS WITH CREAMY HORSERADISH GARLIC SAUCE

Serves: 4 • Serving Size: 3 ounces beef plus 1 tablespoon sauce

Exchanges/Choices

3 Lean Meat
1/2 Fat

Calories	160	
Calories from Fat	45	
Total Fat	5.0	g
Saturated Fat	1.8	g
Trans Fat	0.2	g
Cholesterol	45	mg
Sodium	110	mg
Total Carbohydrate	3	g
Dietary Fiber	0	g
Sugars	1	g
Protein	23	g

1 pound (about 3/4-inch thick) boneless sirloin steak, cut into 4 pieces
1/2 teaspoon coarsely ground black pepper

Sauce

3 tablespoons fat-free sour cream
1 tablespoon reduced-fat mayonnaise
1 teaspoon prepared horseradish
1/2 teaspoon Dijon mustard
1/4 teaspoon Worcestershire sauce
1/2 medium garlic clove, minced

1. Sprinkle both sides of the beef with black pepper (and 1/4 teaspoon salt, if desired).

2. Place a large nonstick skillet over medium-high heat until hot. Coat skillet with cooking spray and cook the beef 4 minutes on each side or to desired doneness. Do not overcook or it will be tough.

3. Meanwhile, in a small bowl, combine the remaining sauce ingredients. Serve alongside the steaks.

SIRLOIN STEAKS AU JUS

Serves: 4 • Serving Size: 3 ounces cooked beef plus 1 1/2 teaspoons sauce

1	pound (about 3/4-inch thick) boneless sirloin steak, cut into 4 pieces
1/2	teaspoon chili powder
1/3	cup water
1	teaspoon Worcestershire sauce

1. Sprinkle both sides of the beef with the chili powder. Place a medium nonstick skillet over medium-high heat until hot. Coat skillet with cooking spray. Cook the steaks 4 minutes on each side or until desired doneness in center.

2. Meanwhile, combine the remaining ingredients in a small bowl and set aside.

3. Place the steaks on a plate. Add the Worcestershire mixture to the skillet and bring to a boil over medium-high heat, boil 2 minutes or until reduced to 2 tablespoons. Drizzle evenly over the steaks. Season lightly with salt and pepper, if desired.

Exchanges/Choices

3 Lean Meat

Calories	135
Calories from Fat	40
Total Fat	4.5 g
Saturated Fat	1.6 g
Trans Fat	0.1 g
Cholesterol	40 mg
Sodium	65 mg
Total Carbohydrate	0 g
Dietary Fiber	0 g
Sugars	0 g
Protein	22 g

Cook's Note

These go great over 2 cups of mashed potatoes or brown rice.

GREEN PEPPER STEAK STIR FRY

Serves: 4 • Serving Size: 1 cup beef mixture

Exchanges/Choices

2 Vegetable
2 Lean Meat
1/2 Fat

Calories	180	
Calories from Fat	55	
Total Fat	6.0	g
Saturated Fat	1.4	g
Trans Fat	0.1	g
Cholesterol	30	mg
Sodium	470	mg
Total Carbohydrate	12	g
Dietary Fiber	2	g
Sugars	8	g
Protein	19	g

Sauce

- 1 tablespoon sugar
- 3 tablespoons lite soy sauce
- 2 tablespoons balsamic vinegar
- 1/4 teaspoon dried red pepper flakes

- 2 teaspoons canola oil
- 12 ounces trimmed boneless sirloin steak, thinly sliced
- 2 medium green bell peppers, cut in thin strips
- 1 medium onion, cut in thin strips

1. Stir together the sugar, soy sauce, vinegar, and pepper flakes in a small bowl and set aside.

2. Heat 1 teaspoon of the oil in a large nonstick skillet over medium-high heat until hot. Cook the beef 2 to 3 minutes or until just brown, stirring frequently, using 2 utensils to toss. Set aside on separate plate, covered to keep warm.

4. Heat the remaining teaspoon oil and cook the peppers and onions 4 minutes or until just tender crisp. Add the beef and any accumulated juice and cook 30 seconds, stirring constantly. Remove from heat. Spoon soy mixture evenly over all.

MEXICAN BEEF PATTIES

Serves: 4 • Serving Size: 3 ounces cooked beef and about 1 tablespoon sauce

1	pound 96% extra-lean ground beef
1/2	cup medium picante sauce
1	teaspoon sugar
1	teaspoon ground cumin
2	tablespoons water
1/4	cup fat-free sour cream (optional)
2	tablespoons chopped cilantro (optional)

1. Combine the beef, 1/4 cup of the picante sauce, sugar, and cumin in a medium bowl and shape into 4 patties.

2. Place a medium nonstick skillet over medium-high heat until hot. Coat skillet with cooking spray, cook the patties 5 minutes, turn patties, reduce heat to medium, and cook 5 minutes or until done.

3. Meanwhile, in a small bowl, combine the remaining 1/4 cup picante sauce with the water and set aside.

4. Place patties on serving platter. Add the picante mixture to the pan residue in the skillet and stir and cook 30 seconds to heat thoroughly and blend well. Pour evenly over the patties. Top with sour cream and cilantro, if desired.

Exchanges/Choices

3 Lean Meat

Calories	155	
Calories from Fat	40	
Total Fat	4.5	g
Saturated Fat	2.0	g
Trans Fat	0.0	g
Cholesterol	60	mg
Sodium	340	mg
Total Carbohydrate	3	g
Dietary Fiber	1	g
Sugars	1	g
Protein	24	g

HOMETOWN CHEESEBURGERS

Serves: 4 • Serving Size: 3 ounces cooked beef

Exchanges/Choices

3 Starch

3 Lean Meat

1/2 Fat

Calories	350
Calories from Fat	80
Total Fat	9.0 g
Saturated Fat	3.0 g
Trans Fat	0.5 g
Cholesterol	65 mg
Sodium	560 mg
Total Carbohydrate	40 g
Dietary Fiber	5 g
Sugars	11 g
Protein	31 g

1 pound 96% extra-lean ground beef

2 tablespoons steak sauce

2 tablespoon finely chopped yellow onion

1 medium garlic clove, minced

2 tablespoons chopped parsley leaves

2 slices reduced-fat American cheese, cut in half diagonally

4 whole-wheat hamburger buns, toasted

4 lettuce leaves

1 small tomato, cut in 4 slices

4 small ears corn on the cob, cooked

1. In a medium mixing bowl, combine ground beef, steak sauce, onion, garlic, and parsley. Blend well and form into 4 patties.

2. Place a large nonstick skillet over medium heat until hot. Coat skillet with cooking spray, add beef patties, and cook 4 minutes. Turn patties and cook 4 minutes or until patties are done to your liking.

3. Remove from heat, top beef patties with cheese slices, cover, and let stand 1 minute to allow cheese to melt. Serve on toasted buns with lettuce and tomato slices and corn on the cob on the side.

BURGUNDY MUSHROOM BEEF PATTIES

Serves: 4 • Serving Size: 3 ounces cooked beef and about 1/3 cup mushroom mixture

8	ounces sliced mushrooms
1	pound 96% extra-lean ground beef
1/2	cup dry red wine
1	teaspoon beef bouillon granules
1/2	teaspoon dried oregano leaves

1. Place a large nonstick skillet over medium-high heat until hot. Coat with cooking spray, add mushrooms, coat mushrooms with cooking spray, and cook 5 minutes or until tender, stirring frequently.

2. Meanwhile, shape beef into four patties and set aside.

3. Combine the mushrooms, wine, bouillon granules, and oregano in a medium bowl and set aside.

4. Recoat skillet with cooking spray, reduce heat to medium, add the patties, and cook 4 minutes on each side, or to desired doneness.

5. Place beef patties on serving platter. To pan residue, add the mushroom mixture, increase to medium-high heat, bring to a boil, and continue boiling 1 minute or until reduced slightly. Spoon over beef patties.

Exchanges/Choices

4 Lean Meat

Calories	170	
Calories from Fat	40	
Total Fat	4.5	g
Saturated Fat	2.0	g
Trans Fat	0.3	g
Cholesterol	60	mg
Sodium	315	mg
Total Carbohydrate	3	g
Dietary Fiber	1	g
Sugars	2	g
Protein	26	g

BEEF AND CORN SKILLET CASSEROLE

Serves: 4 • Serving Size: about 3/4 cup beef mixture and 1/2 cup cooked noodles

Exchanges/Choices

2 Starch
3 Lean Meat

Calories	285
Calories from Fat	55
Total Fat	6.0 g
Saturated Fat	2.2 g
Trans Fat	0.3 g
Cholesterol	60 mg
Sodium	490 mg
Total Carbohydrate	33 g
Dietary Fiber	5 g
Sugars	4 g
Protein	29 g

4   ounces uncooked dried no-yolk or whole-wheat egg noodles
1   pound 96% extra-lean ground beef
1   cup frozen corn kernels
3/4 cup water
3/4 cup picante sauce
1   tablespoon chili powder
2   teaspoons sugar

1. Cook noodles according to directions on the package, omitting any salt or oils.

2. Meanwhile, place a large nonstick skillet over medium-high heat until hot, add beef, and cook 3 minutes or until no longer pink, stirring constantly. To beef, add corn, water, picante sauce, and chili powder.

3. Bring to a boil, reduce heat, and simmer, uncovered, 8 minutes or until thickened and most of the liquid has absorbed.

4. Remove from heat, stir in sugar, and season lightly with salt and pepper, if desired. Serve over cooked noodles.

Cook's Note

Adding the sugar at the end cuts the acidity in the dish, while adding the salt at the end gives a more pronounced saltier taste without adding too much sodium to the dish.

WEEKNIGHT MEXICALI BEEF AND RICE

Serves: 4 • Serving Size: 1/4 recipe

1	10-ounce package frozen precooked brown rice
12	ounces 96% extra-lean ground beef
1	14.5-ounce can no-salt-added stewed tomatoes
1/2	1.25-ounce package taco seasoning mix
1	teaspoon ground cumin
1/2	cup finely chopped green onion
1/2	cup fat-free sour cream
1/3	cup shredded reduced-fat sharp cheddar cheese

1. Cook rice according to package directions, omitting any salt or fats.

2. Meanwhile, place a large nonstick skillet over medium-high heat until hot. Add beef and cook 5 to 6 minutes or until no longer pink, stirring occasionally.

3. Add tomatoes, taco seasoning mix, and cumin. Bring to boil, reduce heat, cover tightly, and simmer 5 minutes.

4. Place rice on a serving platter or shallow pasta dish, top with onion, spoon beef mixture evenly over rice, and serve with sour cream and cheddar cheese.

Exchanges/Choices

1 1/2 Starch
2 Vegetable
2 Lean Meat
1/2 Fat

Calories	285	
Calories from Fat	65	
Total Fat	7.0	g
Saturated Fat	3.0	g
Trans Fat	0.2	g
Cholesterol	55	mg
Sodium	545	mg
Total Carbohydrate	33	g
Dietary Fiber	3	g
Sugars	8	g
Protein	25	g

THICK AND BEEFY PINTO BEAN STEW

Serves: 4 • Serving Size: 1 cup

Exchanges/Choices

1 Starch
1 Vegetable
3 Lean Meat

Calories	225
Calories from Fat	30
Total Fat	3.5 g
Saturated Fat	1.4 g
Trans Fat	0.2 g
Cholesterol	40 mg
Sodium	485 mg
Total Carbohydrate	27 g
Dietary Fiber	8 g
Sugars	7 g
Protein	23 g

10 ounces 96% extra-lean ground beef
1 16-ounce can pinto beans, rinsed and drained
1 14.5-ounce can diced tomatoes with zesty mild green chilis
1/2 cup water
1 tablespoon sugar, or pourable sugar substitute
2 teaspoon ground cumin
1/4 cup finely chopped green onion (optional)

1. Place a Dutch oven over medium-high heat until hot. Coat Dutch oven with cooking spray, add beef, and cook 2 to 3 minutes or until no longer pink, stirring constantly. Add the beans, tomatoes, water, sugar, and 1 teaspoon of the cumin, bring to a boil over high heat, reduce heat, cover tightly, and simmer 10 minutes.

2. Remove from heat, stir in remaining 1 teaspoon cumin, and lightly season with salt and pepper, if desired. Serve topped with green onions (optional).

Cook's Note

If time allows, let stand 10 minutes for a more blended flavor.

CHEATER'S SPAGHETTI

Serves: 4 • Serving Size: 1 cup cooked pasta and about 1/2 cup sauce

8 ounces uncooked whole-grain spaghetti noodles
8 ounces 96% extra-lean ground beef
2 medium garlic cloves, minced
1 1/2 cups bottled spaghetti sauce
1/4 cup dry red wine
1 tablespoon dried basil leaves, crumbled
1 teaspoon sugar
2 teaspoons extra virgin olive oil (optional)
1 tablespoon plus 1 teaspoon grated Parmesan cheese

1. Cook pasta according to package directions, omitting any salt or fats.

2. Meanwhile, place a large nonstick skillet over medium-high heat until hot. Coat skillet with cooking spray and cook beef until browned, stirring constantly. Add the garlic, cook 15 seconds, stirring constantly, and add spaghetti sauce, wine, basil, sugar, and oil. Simmer 3 minutes.

3. Serve over drained pasta and top with Parmesan.

Exchanges/Choices

3 Starch
2 Lean Meat

Calories	340
Calories from Fat	40
Total Fat	4.5 g
Saturated Fat	1.6 g
Trans Fat	0.1 g
Cholesterol	30 mg
Sodium	495 mg
Total Carbohydrate	50 g
Dietary Fiber	8 g
Sugars	8 g
Protein	23 g

Cook's Note

Adding the olive oil at the end gives a richness that would be lost if added earlier.

HAMBURGER ROUNDUP

Serves: 4 • Serving Size: about 1 1/4 cups

Exchanges/Choices

1 1/2 Starch
1 Vegetable
3 Lean Meat

Calories	275	
Calories from Fat	45	
Total Fat	5.0	g
Saturated Fat	2.1	g
Trans Fat	0.3	g
Cholesterol	60	mg
Sodium	315	mg
Total Carbohydrate	29	g
Dietary Fiber	3	g
Sugars	5	g
Protein	29	g

4 ounces uncooked whole-grain elbow or rotini pasta
1 pound 96% extra-lean ground beef
8 ounces frozen pepper-onion stir-fry, thawed
1/3 cup ketchup

1. Cook pasta according to package directions, omitting any salt or fats.

2. Meanwhile, heat a large nonstick skillet over high heat. Coat skillet with cooking spray, add beef, and cook 3 minutes or until no longer pink, stirring frequently. Add stir-fry and cook 3 minutes or until onions are tender, stirring constantly. Stir in ketchup, remove skillet from heat, and cover to keep warm.

3. When pasta is cooked, drain well, reserving 1/4 cup of the pasta water. Add the drained pasta and reserved pasta water to the beef mixture and stir until well blended. Season lightly with salt and pepper, if desired.

SEAFOOD ENTREES

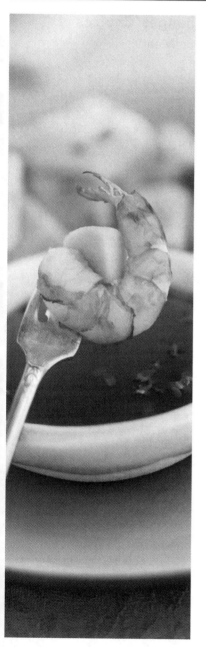

WHITE WINE AND TARRAGON SCALLOPS

Serves: 4 • Serving Size: 1/4 recipe

3/4 teaspoon dried tarragon leaves
1/4 teaspoon paprika
1/4 to 1/2 teaspoon black pepper
1 1/2 pounds scallops, rinsed and patted dry
1 tablespoon extra virgin olive oil
1 tablespoon margarine
1/2 cup dry white wine
2 tablespoons lemon juice
2 tablespoon chopped parsley leaves, or finely chopped green onion

1. In a small bowl, combine tarragon, paprika, and pepper. Mix well

2. Sprinkle scallops evenly with the tarragon mixture.

3. Place a large nonstick skillet over medium-high heat until hot. Add oil and margarine. When margarine has melted, add half the scallops and cook 3 minutes. Turn and cook 2 minutes longer or until scallops are opaque in center, using 2 utensils to turn scallops easily.

4. Remove scallops from skillet and set aside on serving platter. Cover to keep warm and repeat with remaining scallops.

5. Add wine to pan residue, increase heat to high, and boil 45 seconds, scraping bottom and sides of pan. Remove pan from heat, add lemon juice to wine sauce, and spoon over scallops. Sprinkle scallops with parsley and serve.

Exchanges/Choices

4 Lean Meat
1/2 Fat

Calories	215	
Calories from Fat	65	
Total Fat	7.0	g
Saturated Fat	1.3	g
Trans Fat	0.0	g
Cholesterol	70	mg
Sodium	365	mg
Total Carbohydrate	1	g
Dietary Fiber	0	g
Sugars	0	g
Protein	30	g

CAJUN SHRIMP AND PEPPER PASTA

Serves: 4 • Serving Size: about 1 1/4 cups

Exchanges/Choices

1 1/2 Starch
1 Vegetable
2 Lean Meat

Calories	240
Calories from Fat	35
Total Fat	4.0 g
Saturated Fat	1.2 g
Trans Fat	0.0 g
Cholesterol	160 mg
Sodium	580 mg
Total Carbohydrate	27 g
Dietary Fiber	4 g
Sugars	3 g
Protein	23 g

4 ounces uncooked whole-grain vermicelli pasta, broken in half, or rotini
1 pound shrimp, raw, peeled, and deveined
1 cup sliced onions
1 cup sliced red bell peppers
2 teaspoons seafood seasoning (such as Old Bay)
2 medium garlic cloves, minced
2 tablespoons diet margarine
1/4 cup fat-free half and half

1. Cook pasta according to package directions, omitting any salt or fats. Add the shrimp during the last 4 minutes of cooking.

2. Meanwhile, place a large nonstick skillet over medium-high heat until hot. Coat skillet with cooking spray, add the onions and peppers, coat the vegetables with cooking spray, cook 4 minutes or until onions are translucent, stirring frequently. Add the garlic and cook 15 seconds, stirring constantly. Remove from heat, stir in the margarine and half and half, cover, and set aside.

3. Drain pasta and shrimp, add to the onion mixture in the skillet and toss until well blended.

SHRIMP PASTA AND KALAMATA TOMATO TOPPING

Serves: 4 • Serving Size: about 1 1/2 cups

4 ounces uncooked spaghetti or fettuccine (preferably spinach)

1/2 pound shrimp, raw, peeled, and deveined

2 cups diced plum tomatoes

16 pitted kalamata olives, coarsely chopped

3 tablespoons chopped fresh basil leaves, or 1 tablespoon dried basil leaves

2 medium lemons, halved

1. Cook pasta according to package directions, omitting any salt or fats and adding the shrimp during the last 4 minutes of cooking.

2. Meanwhile, in a medium bowl, combine tomatoes, olives, and basil. Toss to blend thoroughly and set aside.

3. Drain pasta and shrimp in a colander and place on a serving platter or in a pasta bowl. Squeeze lemon over pasta and shrimp, top with tomato mixture. Lightly season with salt and pepper, if desired.

Exchanges/Choices

1 1/2 Starch
1 Vegetable
2 Lean Meat

Calories	200	
Calories from Fat	25	
Total Fat	3.0	g
Saturated Fat	0.5	g
Trans Fat	0.0	g
Cholesterol	110	mg
Sodium	270	mg
Total Carbohydrate	27	g
Dietary Fiber	3	g
Sugars	3	g
Protein	17	g

SHRIMP WITH SMOKY COCKTAIL SAUCE

Serves: 4 • Serving Size: 3 ounces cooked shrimp and about 2 tablespoons sauce

Exchanges/Choices

1/2 Carbohydrate
2 Lean Meat

Calories	110
Calories from Fat	10
Total Fat	1.0 g
Saturated Fat	0.3 g
Trans Fat	0.0 g
Cholesterol	160 mg
Sodium	585 mg
Total Carbohydrate	7 g
Dietary Fiber	0 g
Sugars	5 g
Protein	18 g

1	pound shrimp, raw, peeled, and deveined
1	teaspoon Creole seasoning
1/3	cup ketchup
1	tablespoon bottled prepared horseradish
1	tablespoon lemon juice
1	chipotle chili pepper in adobo sauce, chopped and mashed with a fork
1	medium lemon, quartered

1. Place a large nonstick skillet over medium heat until hot. Coat skillet with cooking spray, add shrimp and Creole seasoning, and cook 4 minutes or until opaque in center, stirring frequently. Remove from heat and drain well. Place on a large baking sheet in a single layer and let stand about 5 minutes.

2. Meanwhile, in a small bowl, combine remaining ingredients except lemon.

3. Serve shrimp with sauce and lemon wedges.

DELICATE CRAB FRITTATA

Serves: 4 • Serving Size: 1/4 frittata

1 1/2 cups (equal to 6 eggs) egg substitute

1/3 cup evaporated fat-free milk

1/8 teaspoon cayenne pepper

2 6-ounce cans white crab meat, lightly rinsed and drained in a fine mesh strainer

1/2 cup finely chopped green bell pepper

1/4 cup finely chopped green onion

1/2 cup shredded reduced-fat sharp cheddar cheese

1. In a small mixing bowl, combine egg substitute, evaporated milk, and cayenne and whisk until smooth. Lightly season with salt and black pepper. Stir in crab and green pepper.

2. Place a large nonstick skillet over medium heat. Coat skillet with cooking spray. Add egg mixture, cover, and cook 10 minutes or until just slightly moist on top.

3. Remove from heat and sprinkle with salt (optional), green onion, and cheese. Cover and let stand 3 minutes to allow cheese to melt and flavors to develop. Cut into 4 wedges and serve.

Exchanges/Choices

1/2 Carbohydrate

3 Lean Meat

Calories	150	
Calories from Fat	30	
Total Fat	3.5	g
Saturated Fat	2.0	g
Trans Fat	0.0	g
Cholesterol	65	mg
Sodium	575	mg
Total Carbohydrate	7	g
Dietary Fiber	0	g
Sugars	4	g
Protein	22	g

SPICY SOY TUNA STEAKS

Serves: 4 • Serving Size: 3 ounces cooked tuna

Exchanges/Choices

4 Lean Meat

Calories	165	
Calories from Fat	45	
Total Fat	5.0	g
Saturated Fat	1.4	g
Trans Fat	0.0	g
Cholesterol	40	mg
Sodium	280	mg
Total Carbohydrate	1	g
Dietary Fiber	0	g
Sugars	1	g
Protein	26	g

2 tablespoons lite soy sauce
1 tablespoon balsamic vinegar
1/8 to 1/4 teaspoon dried red pepper flakes
4 4-ounce tuna steaks

1. Stir together the soy sauce, vinegar, and pepper flakes in a small bowl. Place the tuna on a dinner plate, spoon all but 1 tablespoon of the mixture evenly over the tuna. Turn tuna over several times to coat evenly and let stand 5 minutes.

2. Heat a grill pan coated with cooking spray over high heat. Cook tuna 2 minutes on each side or until very pink in center (discard marinade on plate).

3. Place the tuna on serving platter and drizzle the reserved tablespoon soy sauce mixture over all. Season with black pepper, if desired.

Cook's Note

It is very important not to overcook the tuna or it will become dry and tough.

SALMON FILLETS WITH PINEAPPLE SALSA

Serves: 4 • Serving Size: 3 ounces cooked fillet and about 1/2 cup salsa

4 4-ounce salmon fillets, rinsed and patted dry

1/2 teaspoon dried thyme leaves

Salsa

1 15.25-ounce can pineapple tidbits, packed in juice, drained

1/2 cup finely chopped red bell pepper

1/4 cup finely chopped red onion

1 teaspoon grated ginger

1/8 teaspoon dried red pepper flakes (optional)

1. Preheat broiler.

2. Line a baking sheet with foil, coat with cooking spray, and place the salmon, skin side down, on baking sheet. Sprinkle fish with thyme and season lightly with salt and pepper, if desired. Broil 10 minutes or until fish flakes.

3. Meanwhile, in a small bowl, combine all salsa ingredients and set aside.

4. Serve the salmon with the salsa alongside.

Exchanges/Choices

1 Fruit

4 Lean Meat

1/2 Fat

Calories	255
Calories from Fat	90
Total Fat	10.0 g
Saturated Fat	1.8 g
Trans Fat	0.0 g
Cholesterol	80 mg
Sodium	60 mg
Total Carbohydrate	15 g
Dietary Fiber	2 g
Sugars	12 g
Protein	26 g

NO-FRY FISH FRY

Serves: 4 • Serving Size: 3-ounce cooked fillet

Exchanges/Choices

3 Lean Meat

Calories	130	
Calories from Fat	20	
Total Fat	2.5	g
Saturated Fat	0.8	g
Trans Fat	0.0	g
Cholesterol	50	mg
Sodium	180	mg
Total Carbohydrate	4	g
Dietary Fiber	0	g
Sugars	0	g
Protein	23	g

2 tablespoons yellow cornmeal

2 teaspoons Cajun seasoning

4 4-ounce tilapia fillets, or any mild lean white fish, rinsed and patted dry

Lemon wedges (optional)

1. Preheat broiler.

2. Coat a broiler rack and pan with cooking spray and set aside.

3. Place the cornmeal and Cajun seasoning in a shallow pan, such as a pie pan, and mix thoroughly to blend. Coat each fillet with cooking spray and coat evenly with the cornmeal mixture. Place on broiler rack and broil 6 inches away from heat source for 3 minutes on each side.

4. Remove from heat, season lightly with salt and pepper, if desired, and serve with lemon wedges, if desired. Serve immediately for peak flavors and texture.

FISH FILLETS WITH TOMATO-CAPER SALSA

Serves: 4 • Serving Size: 3 ounces cooked fish and 1/3 cup salsa

4 4-ounce tilapia fillets, or any lean mild white fish, rinsed and patted dry

Paprika to taste

1 medium lemon, quartered

Salsa

5 ounces sweet grape cherry tomatoes, quartered

12 pitted kalamata olives, coarsely chopped

1/4 cup capers, drained

1/4 cup chopped parsley

1/2 medium garlic clove, minced

1. Place a large nonstick skillet over medium heat until hot. Coat skillet with cooking spray. Sprinkle both sides of each fillet evenly with paprika, and lightly season with salt and pepper, if desired. Cook 3 minutes, turn, and cook 2 to 3 minutes longer or until opaque in center.

2. Meanwhile, combine the salsa ingredients in a small bowl.

3. To serve, place fillets on a serving platter, squeeze lemon evenly over all, and spoon equal amounts of the salsa on each fillet.

Exchanges/Choices

3 Lean Meat

Calories	135
Calories from Fat	30
Total Fat	3.5 g
Saturated Fat	1.0 g
Trans Fat	0.0 g
Cholesterol	50 mg
Sodium	410 mg
Total Carbohydrate	4 g
Dietary Fiber	1 g
Sugars	1 g
Protein	23 g

FISH FILLETS WITH LEMON PARSLEY TOPPING

Serves: 4 • Serving Size: about 4 1/2 ounces cooked fish and 1 tablespoon parsley mixture

Exchanges/Choices

5 Lean Meat
1 1/2 Fat

Calories	285	
Calories from Fat	155	
Total Fat	17.0	g
Saturated Fat	3.0	g
Trans Fat	0.0	g
Cholesterol	75	mg
Sodium	75	mg
Total Carbohydrate	1	g
Dietary Fiber	0	g
Sugars	0	g
Protein	33	g

4 6-ounce lean white fish fillets (such as tilapia, snapper, or flounder), rinsed and patted dry
   Paprika to taste
1/4 cup extra virgin olive oil
1/2 teaspoon grated lemon zest
2 tablespoons finely chopped parsley
1/4 teaspoon dried dill weed
1 medium lemon, halved

1. Preheat oven to 400°F.

2. Line a baking sheet with foil, coat foil with cooking spray, arrange the fillets on foil, and sprinkle evenly with the paprika. Season lightly with salt and pepper, if desired. Bake 10 minutes or until fish is opaque in center.

3. While fish is cooking, combine the remaining ingredients, except lemon halves, in a small mixing bowl and set aside.

4. Using a slotted spatula, remove the fish, place on four dinner plates, and squeeze lemon juice evenly over all. Top with the parsley mixture.

CAYENNE-BUTTERED FISH

Serves: 4 • Serving Size: 3 ounces fish and about 2 teaspoons margarine mixture

4   4-ounce lean mild fish fillets (such as flounder), rinsed and patted dry
1/2   teaspoon chili powder
2   tablespoons diet margarine
2   teaspoons Dijon mustard
1/8   teaspoon cayenne

1. Preheat oven to 400°F.

2. Coat a nonstick baking sheet with cooking spray. Arrange fish fillets on sheet, lightly coat fish with cooking spray, sprinkle evenly with chili powder, and bake 10 minutes or until opaque in center.

3. In a small bowl, combine margarine, mustard, and cayenne, and season lightly with salt and pepper, if desired. Top each fillet with equal amounts of the margarine mixture (about 2 teaspoons per serving).

Exchanges/Choices

3 Lean Meat

Calories	130
Calories from Fat	35
Total Fat	4.0 g
Saturated Fat	1.1 g
Trans Fat	0.0 g
Cholesterol	60 mg
Sodium	200 mg
Total Carbohydrate	1 g
Dietary Fiber	0 g
Sugars	0 g
Protein	21 g

Cook's Note

Spraying the fillets with cooking spray and chili powder helps the chili powder act as a "blender," spreading slightly to give the fillets good color.

POULTRY ENTREES

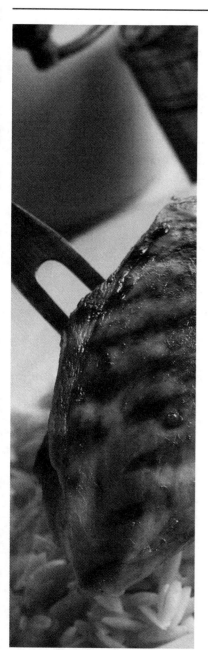

CHICKEN WITH WHITE WINE AND CAPERS

Serves: 4 • Serving Size: 3 ounces cooked chicken plus 1/4 cup sauce

4 4-ounce boneless chicken breasts, rinsed and patted dry, flattened to 1/2-inch thickness

2 teaspoons tomato, basil, and garlic salt-free seasoning blend

1/2 cup dry white wine

2 tablespoons capers, drained

1 cup diced plum tomatoes

1/4 cup chopped green onions

1 teaspoon dried oregano leaves, crumbled

2 teaspoons extra virgin olive oil

1. Sprinkle both sides of chicken with seasoning blend.

2. Place a medium nonstick skillet over medium-high heat until hot. Coat skillet with cooking spray and cook the chicken 3 minutes on each side or until no longer pink in center. Remove from skillet, set aside on separate plate, and cover to keep warm.

3. Add the remaining ingredients, except the oil, to the skillet and bring to a boil. Boil 3 to 4 minutes or until thickened slightly. Remove from heat, then add the oil and 1/4 teaspoon salt, if desired. Spoon evenly over the chicken.

Exchanges/Choices
4 Lean Meat

Calories	180
Calories from Fat	45
Total Fat	5.0 g
Saturated Fat	1.1 g
Trans Fat	0.0 g
Cholesterol	65 mg
Sodium	190 mg
Total Carbohydrate	3 g
Dietary Fiber	1 g
Sugars	2 g
Protein	25 g

SWEET AND SPICY CHICKEN AND SNOW PEAS

Serves: 4 • Serving Size: 1 1/2 cups

Exchanges/Choices

1/2 Carbohydrate
1 Vegetable
3 Lean Meat

Calories	200
Calories from Fat	25
Total Fat	3.0 g
Saturated Fat	0.8 g
Trans Fat	0.0 g
Cholesterol	65 mg
Sodium	650 mg
Total Carbohydrate	15 g
Dietary Fiber	2 g
Sugars	11 g
Protein	28 g

1 pound boneless chicken breasts, thinly sliced
1 cup presliced peppers and onions, or 1/2 cup sliced peppers and 1/2 cup sliced onions
1 cup matchstick carrots
6 ounces fresh or frozen and thawed snow peas
1/4 cup lite soy sauce
2 tablespoons cider vinegar
2 tablespoons sugar, or pourable sugar substitute
1/8 teaspoon dried red pepper flakes
1 tablespoon sesame seeds, toasted (optional)

1. Place a large nonstick skillet over medium-high heat until hot. Coat the skillet with cooking spray, add chicken, and cook 2 minutes or until no longer pink in center, stirring constantly. Set aside.

2. Recoat the skillet with cooking spray, add the peppers, onions, and carrots, coat vegetables with cooking spray, and cook 3 minutes, stirring occasionally. Add the snow peas, coat with cooking spray, and cook 2 minutes or until tender crisp. Add the chicken and toss.

3. Meanwhile, combine remaining ingredients, except sesame seeds, in a small bowl.

4. To serve, place equal amounts of the chicken mixture in four shallow bowls. Spoon equal amounts of the soy mixture over each serving and sprinkle evenly with sesame seeds.

Cook's Note

For an even faster dish, skip the first step and use 2 cups cooked chicken, adding it at the end.

EASY SEASONED SKILLET CHICKEN

Serves: 4 • Serving Size: 3 ounces cooked chicken

4 4-ounce boneless chicken breasts, rinsed and patted dry, flattened to 1/2-inch thickness

1/2 teaspoon dried tarragon or oregano leaves, crumbled

2 tablespoons lite olive oil vinaigrette

1. Sprinkle the smooth side of the chicken pieces with the tarragon and set aside.

2. Place a large nonstick skillet over medium-high heat until hot. Add 1 tablespoon of the vinaigrette, tilt skillet to coat lightly, cook chicken seasoned-side down for 4 minutes, turn, and cook 3 minutes or until no longer pink in center.

3. Remove from heat and drizzle the remaining 1 tablespoon vinaigrette evenly over all. Cover and let stand 2 minutes to absorb flavors. Place on serving platter and drizzle any pan drippings evenly over all.

Exchanges/Choices

3 Lean Meat

Calories	145
Calories from Fat	35
Total Fat	4.0 g
Saturated Fat	1.0 g
Trans Fat	0.0 g
Cholesterol	65 mg
Sodium	115 mg
Total Carbohydrate	1 g
Dietary Fiber	0 g
Sugars	1 g
Protein	24 g

SWEET AND TANGY SAUCE'D CHICKEN

Serves: 4 • Serving Size: 3 ounces cooked chicken

Exchanges/Choices
1/2 Carbohydrate
3 Lean Meat

Calories	165	
Calories from Fat	25	
Total Fat	3.0	g
Saturated Fat	0.8	g
Trans Fat	0.0	g
Cholesterol	65	mg
Sodium	455	mg
Total Carbohydrate	8	g
Dietary Fiber	0	g
Sugars	7	g
Protein	25	g

2 tablespoons sugar

2 tablespoons Dijon mustard

1 1/2 tablespoons lite soy sauce

4 4-ounce boneless skinless chicken breast halves, rinsed and patted dry, flattened to 1/4-inch thickness

1/4 cup water

1. In a small bowl, combine sugar, mustard, and soy sauce. Stir to blend thoroughly and place 2 tablespoons of the mixture in a separate small bowl.

2. Place a large nonstick skillet over medium heat until hot. Coat skillet with cooking spray. Brush 1 tablespoon of the sauce evenly over the chicken pieces and place sauce-side down in skillet. Cook 3 minutes, brush 1 tablespoon sauce on chicken pieces, turn, and cook 3 minutes or until no longer pink in center. Place chicken on serving platter.

3. Add reserved mustard mixture and water to the skillet, bring to a boil over medium-high heat, and boil 2 minutes or until sauce is thickened slightly and liquid measures 2 tablespoons, scraping the bottom of the skillet with a flat spatula. Spoon sauce over chicken to serve.

CHICKEN WITH ITALIAN SALSA AND FETA

Serves: 4 • Serving Size: 3 ounces cooked chicken and about 1/3 cup salsa and cheese

4 4-ounce boneless chicken breast halves, rinsed and patted dry

1 teaspoon dried oregano leaves

6 ounces uncooked whole-grain rotini

Salsa

1 1/2 cups grape tomatoes, quartered

8 pitted kalamata olives, coarsely chopped

1 teaspoon dried basil leaves

1 medium garlic clove, minced

2 teaspoons extra virgin olive oil

1/4 cup reduced-fat feta, crumbled

1. Sprinkle both sides of the chicken with oregano. Lightly season with black pepper, if desired.

2. Place a large nonstick skillet over medium-high heat. Lightly coat with cooking spray and cook the chicken 5 to 6 minutes on each side or until no longer pink in center.

3. Meanwhile, cook pasta according to package directions, omitting any salt or fats. Combine the salsa ingredients, except the cheese, in a small bowl.

4. Place a bed of pasta on a serving platter and top with the chicken. Spoon the salsa on top of the chicken and sprinkle cheese evenly over all.

Exchanges/Choices

1 Starch
1 Vegetable
4 Lean Meat

Calories	270
Calories from Fat	65
Total Fat	7.0 g
Saturated Fat	1.9 g
Trans Fat	0.0 g
Cholesterol	70 mg
Sodium	225 mg
Total Carbohydrate	20 g
Dietary Fiber	4 g
Sugars	2 g
Protein	30 g

CAJUN-SAUCE'D CHICKEN

Serves: 4 • Serving Size: 3 ounces cooked chicken and 1 tablespoon sauce

Exchanges/Choices

3 Lean Meat
1 Fat

Calories	190
Calories from Fat	90
Total Fat	10.0 g
Saturated Fat	1.7 g
Trans Fat	0.0 g
Cholesterol	65 mg
Sodium	75 mg
Total Carbohydrate	1 g
Dietary Fiber	0 g
Sugars	0 g
Protein	24 g

1 teaspoon dried thyme leaves
1/2 teaspoon garlic powder
1/2 teaspoon paprika
4 4-ounce boneless chicken breasts, rinsed and patted dry
2 tablespoons extra virgin olive oil
1/3 cup water
2 tablespoons lemon juice
2 teaspoons Louisiana hot sauce

1. Combine the thyme, garlic powder, and paprika in a small bowl and sprinkle evenly over both sides of the chicken, pressing down lightly with your fingertips to adhere.

2. Heat 1 teaspoon of the oil in a large nonstick skillet over medium-high heat. Cook the chicken 5 to 6 minutes on each side or until no longer pink in center. Set aside on serving platter.

3. Add the water and lemon juice to the pan residue in the skillet and bring to a boil over medium-high heat, stirring bottom and sides. Boil 2 to 3 minutes or until reduced to 2 tablespoons liquid. Remove from heat, stir in the hot sauce and remaining oil, and spoon evenly over all. Lightly season with black pepper, if desired.

ARTICHOKES AND ROASTED PEPPER CHICKEN

Serves: 4 • Serving Size: 3 ounces cooked chicken and about 1/3 cup artichoke mixture

2 tablespoons extra virgin olive oil

4 4-ounce boneless chicken breasts, rinsed and patted dry

1/2 13.75-ounce can quartered artichoke hearts, drained

2 medium garlic cloves, minced

1/2 cup chopped roasted peppers

2 tablespoons chopped fresh basil leaves, or 2 teaspoons dried basil leaves

1. Heat 1 teaspoon of the oil in a large nonstick skillet over medium-high heat. Cook the chicken 5 to 6 minutes on each side or until no longer pink in center. Place on serving platter, and cover to keep warm.

2. Add 1 tablespoon of the oil to the pan residue in the skillet. Cook the artichokes and garlic 1 minute, stirring constantly. Stir in the peppers and basil and cook 15 seconds. Spoon over chicken and drizzle with the remaining oil.

Exchanges/Choices

1 Vegetable
3 Lean Meat
1 Fat

Calories	210
Calories from Fat	90
Total Fat	10.0 g
Saturated Fat	1.7 g
Trans Fat	0.0 g
Cholesterol	65 mg
Sodium	225 mg
Total Carbohydrate	4 g
Dietary Fiber	1 g
Sugars	1 g
Protein	25 g

CREAMY CHICKEN WITH ROSEMARY

Serves: 4 • Serving Size: 3 ounces cooked chicken and about 1/2 cup sauce

Exchanges/Choices

1 1/2 Starch
1/2 Carbohydrate
4 Lean Meat

Calories	330
Calories from Fat	65
Total Fat	7.0 g
Saturated Fat	3.2 g
Trans Fat	0.0 g
Cholesterol	80 mg
Sodium	430 mg
Total Carbohydrate	34 g
Dietary Fiber	3 g
Sugars	4 g
Protein	30 g

2 cups frozen precooked brown rice
8 (about 1 pound total) chicken tenderloins
1 10.75-ounce can reduced-fat cream of chicken soup
6 tablespoons light sour cream
4 medium green onions, chopped
1/4 to 1/2 teaspoon dried rosemary leaves, crumbled

1. Prepare rice according to the package directions, omitting any salt or fats.

2. In a medium mixing bowl, combine soup, sour cream, all but 2 tablespoons of the onions, and the rosemary. Set aside.

3. Place a large nonstick skillet over medium-high heat until hot. Coat skillet with cooking spray, add chicken, and cook 1 to 2 minutes or until lightly browned. Turn pieces over and spoon the soup mixture evenly over all.

4. Bring to a boil, reduce heat, cover tightly, and simmer 10 minutes or until chicken is no longer pink in center, stirring midway. Top with remaining green onions and serve over rice.

Cook's Note

This recipe is also great served over 2 cups of no-yolk egg noodles.

CHICKEN WITH QUICK CUPBOARD GRAVY

Serves: 4 • Serving Size: 3 ounces cooked chicken and about 1/3 cup gravy

4 4-ounce boneless, skinless chicken breasts, rinsed and patted dry

Paprika to taste

1 12-ounce jar chicken gravy

1 1/2 teaspoons Dijon mustard

3/4 teaspoon dried thyme leaves

1. Sprinkle one side of the chicken breasts with paprika.

2. Heat a large nonstick skillet over medium-high heat until hot. Coat skillet with cooking spray, add the chicken seasoned-side down, and cook 2 minutes to brown lightly on one side.

3. Meanwhile, whisk together the gravy, mustard, and thyme in a small bowl.

4. Turn the chicken, spoon the gravy mixture over the chicken, cover tightly, reduce heat, and simmer 10 minutes or until chicken is no longer pink in center.

Exchanges/Choices

1/2 Starch
3 Lean Meat

Calories	175	
Calories from Fat	55	
Total Fat	6.0	g
Saturated Fat	1.5	g
Trans Fat	0.0	g
Cholesterol	70	mg
Sodium	455	mg
Total Carbohydrate	5	g
Dietary Fiber	0	g
Sugars	0	g
Protein	24	g

PIZZA SAUCE'D CHICKEN

Serves: 4 • Serving Size: 3 ounces cooked chicken

Exchanges/Choices

1 1/2 Starch

4 Lean Meat

Calories	290
Calories from Fat	55
Total Fat	6.0 g
Saturated Fat	2.4 g
Trans Fat	0.0 g
Cholesterol	80 mg
Sodium	330 mg
Total Carbohydrate	24 g
Dietary Fiber	4 g
Sugars	2 g
Protein	33 g

4 ounces uncooked whole-grain spaghetti

4 4-ounce boneless, skinless chicken breast halves, rinsed and patted dry

1/3 cup bottled or canned pizza sauce

1 1/2 teaspoons dried basil leaves

1/4 teaspoon dried red pepper flakes (optional)

8 turkey pepperoni slices, halved

1/2 cup shredded part-skim mozzarella cheese

4 teaspoons grated Parmesan cheese

1. Cook pasta according to package directions, omitting any salt or fats.

2. Heat a medium nonstick skillet over medium-high heat until hot. Coat skillet with cooking spray. Cook chicken 5 to 6 minutes on each side or until no longer pink in center.

3. Meanwhile, combine the pizza sauce, basil leaves, and pepper flakes in a small bowl and set aside.

4. Spoon equal amounts of the pizza sauce mixture on each chicken piece. Sprinkle evenly with the pepperoni pieces and top with the cheeses. Cover and cook 1 minute or until cheese begins to melt slightly. Serve over pasta.

SKILLET CHICKEN WITH GREEN CHILIS AND CILANTRO

Serves: 4 • Serving Size: 3 ounces cooked chicken

4	4-ounce boneless, skinless chicken breast halves, rinsed and patted dry
3/4	teaspoon ground cumin
1	medium lime, halved crosswise
1	4-ounce can chopped green chilis
1/4	cup shredded part-skim mozzarella cheese, or shredded reduced-fat sharp cheddar cheese
1/4	cup chopped cilantro leaves
1	small tomato, seeded and diced

1. Sprinkle one side of the chicken with cumin.

2. Place a large nonstick skillet over medium-high heat until hot. Coat skillet with cooking spray, add the chicken seasoned-side down, and cook 2 minutes to brown lightly on one side. Turn chicken, squeeze the juice of one of the lime halves evenly over the chicken, spoon the green chilis evenly over all, cover, reduce heat, and simmer 10 minutes or until chicken is no longer pink in center.

3. Remove from heat, place on serving platter, and sprinkle evenly with the cheese, cilantro, and tomatoes. Cut the remaining lime half into 4 wedges to serve with chicken.

Exchanges/Choices
4 Lean Meat

Calories	160	
Calories from Fat	35	
Total Fat	4.0	g
Saturated Fat	1.5	g
Trans Fat	0.0	g
Cholesterol	70	mg
Sodium	175	mg
Total Carbohydrate	3	g
Dietary Fiber	1	g
Sugars	1	g
Protein	26	g

GRILLED CHICKEN WITH ASIAN-GINGER SAUCE

Serves: 4 • Serving Size: 3 ounces cooked chicken and 1 tablespoon sauce

Exchanges/Choices

4 Lean Meat

Calories	180	
Calories from Fat	55	
Total Fat	6.0	g
Saturated Fat	1.0	g
Trans Fat	0.0	g
Cholesterol	65	mg
Sodium	345	mg
Total Carbohydrate	4	g
Dietary Fiber	0	g
Sugars	4	g
Protein	25	g

1 tablespoon sugar

2 tablespoons lite soy sauce

2 tablespoons cider vinegar

1 tablespoon canola oil

1 to 2 teaspoons grated ginger

4 4-ounce boneless skinless chicken breasts, rinsed and patted dry

1 teaspoon coarsely ground black pepper

1. Whisk together the sugar, soy sauce, vinegar, oil, and ginger in a small bowl. Reserve 2 tablespoons of the mixture in a separate small bowl.

2. Sprinkle both sides of the chicken with the black pepper, pressing down lightly with your fingertips to adhere.

3. Lightly coat a grill pan or nonstick skillet with cooking spray and place over medium-high heat. Using the 2 tablespoons of reserved sauce, brush 1 tablespoon on the chicken and cook 5 to 6 minutes. Turn, brush with the remaining tablespoon, and cook an additional 5 to 6 minutes or until no longer pink in center.

4. Place on serving platter and spoon remaining sauce evenly over all.

Cook's Note

You can serve this as is, or make 2 cups cooked brown rice tossed with 2 tablespoons finely chopped green onion, divided into 1/2-cup servings, to catch the sauce.

CHICKEN TENDERS WITH SPICY TOMATO AND BLACK BEANS

Serves: 4 • Serving Size: 3 ounces cooked chicken, 1/2 cup bean mixture, and 2 tablespoons sour cream

12 (about 1 1/4 pounds total) chicken tenders
1/2 teaspoon chili powder
1 10-ounce can mild diced tomatoes and green chilis
1/2 15.5-ounce can no-salt-added black beans, rinsed and drained
2 teaspoons extra virgin olive oil
1/2 cup fat-free sour cream

1. Sprinkle both sides of the chicken pieces evenly with chili powder.

2. Place a large nonstick skillet over medium-high heat until hot. Coat skillet with cooking spray, cook chicken 2 minutes or until browned on one side, turn, and top with the tomatoes and beans. Bring to a boil (over medium-high heat), and cook 3 minutes or until chicken is no longer pink in the center.

3. Remove from heat and drizzle the oil evenly over all. Serve in shallow soup bowls, topped with sour cream.

Exchanges/Choices

1/2 Starch
1/2 Carbohydrate
4 Lean Meat

Calories	265
Calories from Fat	55
Total Fat	6.0 g
Saturated Fat	1.5 g
Trans Fat	0.0 g
Cholesterol	85 mg
Sodium	405 mg
Total Carbohydrate	16 g
Dietary Fiber	3 g
Sugars	4 g
Protein	35 g

QUICK COMFORT CHICKEN AND RICE

Serves: 4 • Serving Size: 1 cup

Exchanges/Choices

2 Starch

3 Lean Meat

Calories	295
Calories from Fat	65
Total Fat	7.0 g
Saturated Fat	2.5 g
Trans Fat	0.0 g
Cholesterol	60 mg
Sodium	570 mg
Total Carbohydrate	32 g
Dietary Fiber	3 g
Sugars	3 g
Protein	25 g

1 1/4 cups water
3/4 cup uncooked quick-cooking brown rice
1 teaspoon dried thyme leaves
1/8 teaspoon cayenne pepper
7 light spreadable Swiss cheese wedges
1 1/2 cups cooked diced chicken breast meat
1/2 cup frozen green peas, thawed
1 2-ounce jar diced pimiento
1/4 cup chopped parsley, or green onion

1. Bring the water to a boil over high heat in a large saucepan. Stir in the rice, thyme, and cayenne, reduce heat, cover, and simmer 10 to 12 minutes or until water is absorbed.

2. Stir in the cheese until melted. Gently stir in the remaining ingredients.

CHICKEN AND VEGETABLE MACARONI AND CHEESE

Serves: 7 • Serving Size: 1 cup

1 7.25-ounce box macaroni and cheese dinner

1 8-ounce package frozen broccoli and cauliflower mixture, thawed

4 ounces frozen red pepper stir-fry, thawed, or 4-ounce jar sliced pimiento

1/4 cup evaporated fat-free milk

2 tablespoons reduced-fat margarine

9 ounces frozen precooked diced chicken breast meat, thawed according to package directions

1. Cook pasta in boiling water, omitting any salt or fats, for 6 minutes or until almost tender. Add broccoli mixture and peppers to pasta, return to a boil, and boil 2 minutes or until vegetables are just tender-crisp.

2. Drain pasta and vegetables and return to pot. Add cheese mix, milk, and margarine and stir until just blended, using a rubber spatula. Add chicken and, if desired, salt and stir to blend thoroughly. Serve immediately.

Exchanges/Choices

1 Starch
1 Vegetable
2 Lean Meat

Calories	190
Calories from Fat	35
Total Fat	4.0 g
Saturated Fat	1.7 g
Trans Fat	0.0 g
Cholesterol	35 mg
Sodium	430 mg
Total Carbohydrate	25 g
Dietary Fiber	2 g
Sugars	5 g
Protein	14 g

SMOKED TURKEY SAUSAGE AND PEPPERS ON TOASTED PUMPERNICKEL

Serves: 4 • Serving Size: 1 sandwich

Exchanges/Choices

1 Starch
1/2 Carbohydrate
1 Vegetable
2 Lean Meat
1/2 Fat

Calories	255
Calories from Fat	70
Total Fat	8.0 g
Saturated Fat	2.2 g
Trans Fat	0.0 g
Cholesterol	45 mg
Sodium	880 mg
Total Carbohydrate	28 g
Dietary Fiber	3 g
Sugars	8 g
Protein	13 g

8 ounces lean smoked turkey sausage
2 cups thinly sliced yellow onions
1 cup thinly sliced green bell pepper
3 tablespoons reduced-fat mayonnaise
1 teaspoon prepared mustard
2 teaspoons honey
1/4 cup water
4 dark pumpernickel bread slices, toasted

1. Cut sausage in half lengthwise, then cut each half in fourths crosswise, forming 8 pieces.

2. Place a large nonstick skillet over medium-high heat until hot. Coat skillet with cooking spray, add sausage, and cook 1 minute. Add onion and bell pepper, coat with cooking spray, and cook 4 minutes or until onion is lightly brown, stirring frequently.

3. Meanwhile, in a small bowl, combine mayonnaise, mustard, and honey and stir until well blended. Set aside.

4. Add water to sausage and vegetable mixture and cook 1 minute or until most of the liquid has evaporated, mixing in sausage drippings from the pan bottom as you stir.

5. Remove from heat, spread 1 tablespoon of the mayonnaise mixture evenly over each bread slice, and top with sausage and pepper mixture.

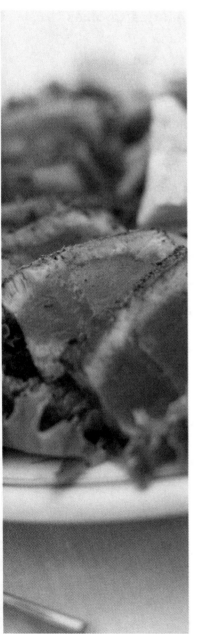

PORK ENTREES

SWEET SPICED ORANGE PORK

Serves: 4 • Serving Size: 3 ounces cooked pork

4 4-ounce boneless center-cut pork chops, trimmed of fat

1 teaspoon ground cinnamon

1 tablespoon lite soy sauce

1 tablespoon plus 1 teaspoon sugar

1 tablespoon cider vinegar

1 teaspoon grated orange zest

1/8 teaspoon dried red pepper flakes (optional)

1. Place a large nonstick skillet over medium-high heat until hot. Coat the skillet with cooking spray. Sprinkle both sides of pork with cinnamon and 1/4 teaspoon salt, if desired. Cook pork 5 minutes on each side or until barely pink in center.

2. Meanwhile, combine the remaining ingredients in a small bowl.

3. Pour sauce evenly over all and cook 30 seconds or until liquid has almost evaporated.

Exchanges/Choices
1/2 Carbohydrate
3 Lean Meat

Calories	175
Calories from Fat	65
Total Fat	7.0 g
Saturated Fat	2.5 g
Trans Fat	0.0 g
Cholesterol	60 mg
Sodium	190 mg
Total Carbohydrate	5 g
Dietary Fiber	0 g
Sugars	4 g
Protein	21 g

ONION PORK CHOPS

Serves: 4 • Serving Size: 1 pork chop and about 2 tablespoons onions

Exchanges/Choices

1 Vegetable

3 Lean Meat

Calories	160
Calories from Fat	55
Total Fat	6.0 g
Saturated Fat	2.1 g
Trans Fat	0.0 g
Cholesterol	60 mg
Sodium	45 mg
Total Carbohydrate	5 g
Dietary Fiber	1 g
Sugars	3 g
Protein	21 g

4 (about 5 ounces each) pork chops with bone in, trimmed of fat

1 medium onion, thinly sliced

2 tablespoons balsamic vinegar

1. Place a large nonstick skillet over medium-high heat until hot. Coat skillet with cooking spray, add pork chops, and cook 2 minutes to brown on one side. Remove and set aside on separate plate.

2. Add the onions, cook 5 minutes or until richly browned, stirring frequently.

3. Place pork (browned side up) and any accumulated juices on top of onions. Sprinkle with 1 tablespoon of the vinegar, reduce heat, cover tightly, and simmer 8 minutes or until pork is no longer pink in center.

4. Remove pork and onions with slotted spatula and place on a serving platter. Add remaining 1 tablespoon vinegar to pan drippings, increase to medium-high heat, and cook 1 minute or until liquid measures 1/4 cup. Pour over pork and onions and season lightly with salt and pepper to taste, if desired.

TENDER COUNTRY PORK CHOPS

Serves: 4 • Serving Size: 3 ounces cooked pork

1/4 cup flour
1 teaspoon paprika
1/2 teaspoon garlic salt
1/2 teaspoon dried thyme leaves
4 (about 1 1/4 pounds total) thin pork chops with bone in
1 tablespoon canola oil

1. In a shallow pan, such as a pie pan, combine flour, paprika, garlic salt, and thyme. Stir to blend thoroughly. Coat pork evenly with flour mixture and place on a separate plate.

2. Place a large nonstick skillet over medium-high heat until hot. Coat skillet with cooking spray, add oil, and tilt skillet to coat bottom evenly. Add pork, immediately reduce heat to medium, cook 4 minutes, and then turn and cook 3 minutes longer or until barely pink in center.

Exchanges/Choices

1/2 Starch
3 Lean Meat
1 Fat

Calories	230	
Calories from Fat	100	
Total Fat	11.0	g
Saturated Fat	2.8	g
Trans Fat	0.0	g
Cholesterol	70	mg
Sodium	210	mg
Total Carbohydrate	6	g
Dietary Fiber	0	g
Sugars	0	g
Protein	26	g

GARLIC PORK CHOPS WITH TARRAGON SAUCE

Serves: 4 • Serving Size: 1 pork chop plus 2 tablespoons sauce

Exchanges/Choices

3 Lean Meat
1 Fat

Calories	195
Calories from Fat	90
Total Fat	10.0 g
Saturated Fat	2.9 g
Trans Fat	0.0 g
Cholesterol	60 mg
Sodium	155 mg
Total Carbohydrate	3 g
Dietary Fiber	0 g
Sugars	2 g
Protein	23 g

4 4-ounce boneless pork chops
1/2 teaspoon garlic powder
Paprika to taste

Sauce
1/2 cup plain fat-free yogurt
1 tablespoon Dijon mustard
1 1/2 teaspoons dried tarragon leaves
2 teaspoons extra virgin olive oil

1. Sprinkle both sides of the pork chops with the garlic powder and lightly season with salt and black pepper, if desired. Sprinkle evenly with the paprika. Place a medium nonstick skillet over medium-high heat until hot. Coat skillet with cooking spray. Cook the pork chops 4 minutes on each side or until barely pink in center.

2. Meanwhile, combine the sauce ingredients and lightly season with salt, if desired, in small bowl and set aside.

3. Serve sauce spooned over each pork chop and sprinkle with additional black pepper.

CUMIN PORK AND SWEET POTATOES WITH SPICED BUTTER

Serves: 4 • Serving Size: 3 ounces cooked pork, 1/2 potato, and about 1 tablespoon topping

2 8-ounce sweet potatoes, pierced in several areas with fork

1/2 teaspoon ground cumin

Paprika to taste

4 4-ounce boneless pork cutlets, trimmed of fat

Topping

2 tablespoons reduced-fat margarine

2 tablespoons packed dark brown sugar

1/2 teaspoon grated orange zest

1/4 teaspoon vanilla, butter, and nut flavoring

1/8 teaspoon ground nutmeg

4 small oranges, quartered

1. Cook potatoes in microwave on HIGH setting for 10 to 11 minutes or until fork tender.

2. Meanwhile, place a large nonstick skillet over medium-high heat until hot. Sprinkle cumin and paprika evenly over pork chops and season lightly with salt and pepper if desired. Cook pork chops 4 minutes on each side or until barely pink in center.

3. In a small bowl, stir together the topping ingredients until well blended.

4. Cut potatoes in half lengthwise, fluff with a fork, and spoon equal amounts topping mixture on each half. Serve with quartered oranges alongside.

Exchanges/Choices

1 Starch
1 Fruit
3 Lean Meat
1 Fat

Calories	335
Calories from Fat	90
Total Fat	10.0 g
Saturated Fat	3.4 g
Trans Fat	0.0 g
Cholesterol	60 mg
Sodium	125 mg
Total Carbohydrate	37 g
Dietary Fiber	5 g
Sugars	22 g
Protein	24 g

JERKED PORK WITH NECTARINE–DRIED CHERRY SALSA

Serves: 4 • Serving Size: 3 ounces pork and about 1/3 cup nectarine mixture

Exchanges/Choices

1 1/2 Fruit
3 Lean Meat

Calories	240
Calories from Fat	65
Total Fat	7.0 g
Saturated Fat	2.6 g
Trans Fat	0.0 g
Cholesterol	60 mg
Sodium	260 mg
Total Carbohydrate	21 g
Dietary Fiber	2 g
Sugars	17 g
Protein	22 g

4 4-ounce boneless pork chops, trimmed of fat
1 tablespoon jerk seasoning
2 medium nectarines, finely chopped
1/3 cup dried cherries or cranberries
2 teaspoons grated orange zest
1/4 cup orange juice
1 teaspoon grated ginger (optional)
1/4 teaspoon dried red pepper flakes

1. Sprinkle the jerk seasoning evenly over both sides of the pork.

2. Place a large nonstick skillet over medium-high heat until hot. Coat skillet with cooking spray and cook the pork 4 minutes on each side or until barely pink in center.

3. Meanwhile, combine the remaining ingredients in a medium bowl.

4. Serve nectarine mixture alongside pork.

SKILLET HAM WITH MILD CURRIED APPLES

Serves: 4 • Serving Size: 2 ounces ham and about 1/3 cup apple mixture

2	medium red apples (preferably Gala), cored and cut into 1/2-inch cubes
1/4	cup chopped dried apricots
2	tablespoons packed dark brown sugar
2	tablespoons water
1/2	teaspoon curry powder
1/4	teaspoon vanilla
1 1/2	teaspoons reduced-fat margarine
8	ounces extra-lean ham, cut into 4 slices

1. In a small saucepan, combine the apples, apricots, sugar, water, and curry powder. Bring to a boil over medium high heat. Reduce heat, cover tightly, and simmer 5 minutes or until apples are just tender, stirring occasionally.

2. Remove from heat, stir in vanilla and margarine, cover tightly, and let stand 5 minutes to allow flavors to blend.

3. Place a large nonstick skillet over medium-high heat until hot. Coat skillet with cooking spray. Working in two batches, cook ham on each side 1 to 2 minutes or until beginning to richly brown.

4. Serve ham slices with apple mixture alongside.

Exchanges/Choices
1 1/2 Fruit
2 Lean Meat

Calories	165
Calories from Fat	25
Total Fat	3.0 g
Saturated Fat	0.7 g
Trans Fat	0.0 g
Cholesterol	30 mg
Sodium	725 mg
Total Carbohydrate	26 g
Dietary Fiber	3 g
Sugars	23 g
Protein	12 g

CHEDDARY HAM AND RICE CASSEROLE

Serves: 4 • Serving Size: 1 cup

Exchanges/Choices

1 1/2 Starch
1 Vegetable
1 Med-Fat Meat

Calories	205
Calories from Fat	55
Total Fat	6.0 g
Saturated Fat	2.3 g
Trans Fat	0.0 g
Cholesterol	25 mg
Sodium	495 mg
Total Carbohydrate	26 g
Dietary Fiber	3 g
Sugars	5 g
Protein	12 g

1 teaspoon canola oil
1 cup finely chopped yellow onion
1/2 cup finely chopped green bell pepper
1 10-ounce package frozen precooked brown rice
1/2 cup frozen green peas, thawed
2/3 cup pre-diced extra-lean ham
1/4 cup chopped fresh parsley
1/8 teaspoon cayenne
1/2 cup shredded reduced-fat cheddar cheese

1. In a Dutch oven, heat oil over medium-high heat until hot. Add onions and peppers, cook 4 minutes or until onions are translucent, stirring frequently. Add the ham and cook 30 seconds.

2. Meanwhile, cook rice in microwave according to directions on package. Remove the Dutch oven from the heat, add the rice to the ham mixture, and stir in parsley and cayenne. Season lightly with salt and pepper, if desired, and sprinkle with the cheese.

RUSTIC CABBAGE AND NOODLES

Serves: 4 • Serving Size: 1 1/2 cups cabbage and noodle mixture

4   ounces uncooked no-yolk egg noodles

8   center-cut bacon slices

2   teaspoons canola oil

6   cups (about 1 pound) coarsely chopped green cabbage, about 1-inch pieces (do not shred)

2   cups chopped yellow onions

4   medium cloves garlic, minced

1. Cook noodles according to package directions, omitting any salt or fat.

2. Meanwhile, heat a large nonstick skillet over medium-high heat. Add bacon and cook until very crisp. Place bacon on paper towels and pat dry. Drain off excess grease from skillet, but do not paper towel dry.

3. Add oil to pan residue in skillet and tilt skillet to coat bottom of pan evenly. Add cabbage, onions, and garlic, and cook 8 minutes until beginning to richly brown, stirring frequently, using two utensils (as you would a stir fry) for easier handling.

4. Remove from heat. Crumble bacon and stir into the cabbage mixture. Lightly season with salt and pepper, if desired. Cover and let stand 3 minutes to develop flavors. Serve over egg noodles.

Exchanges/Choices

1 1/2 Starch

3 Vegetable

1 1/2 Fat

Calories	250
Calories from Fat	70
Total Fat	8.0 g
Saturated Fat	1.9 g
Trans Fat	0.0 g
Cholesterol	15 mg
Sodium	315 mg
Total Carbohydrate	35 g
Dietary Fiber	6 g
Sugars	9 g
Protein	11 g

SIDES

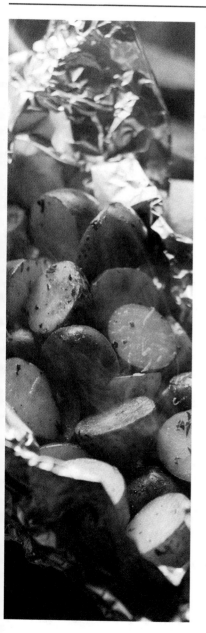

CREAMY DIJON-DILL ASPARAGUS

Serves: 4 • Serving Size: about 5 spears and 2 tablespoons sauce

Sauce

1/3	cup	fat-free sour cream
1	tablespoon	fat-free milk
1	tablespoon	extra virgin olive oil
1	tablespoon	Dijon mustard
1/4	teaspoon	dried dill weed

1/2	cup	water
1	pound	asparagus spears, trimmed

1. Combine the sauce ingredients in a small microwave-safe bowl and set aside.

2. Bring water to a boil in a large nonstick skillet over medium-high heat, add the asparagus, return to a boil, cover tightly, and continue boiling 2 minutes or until just tender-crisp. Drain well and place on serving platter.

3. Place the sauce in the microwave and cook on high setting 15 seconds or until slightly warm. Spoon evenly over the asparagus and season lightly with salt and pepper, if desired.

Exchanges/Choices

1 Vegetable
1 Fat

Calories	65	
Calories from Fat	30	
Total Fat	3.5	g
Saturated Fat	0.6	g
Trans Fat	0.0	g
Cholesterol	0	mg
Sodium	120	mg
Total Carbohydrate	6	g
Dietary Fiber	1	g
Sugars	2	g
Protein	2	g

SESAME-ROASTED ASPARAGUS

Serves: 4 • Serving Size: about 5 spears

Exchanges/Choices

1 Vegetable

Calories	20
Calories from Fat	10
Total Fat	1.0 g
Saturated Fat	0.1 g
Trans Fat	0.0 g
Cholesterol	0 mg
Sodium	10 mg
Total Carbohydrate	3 g
Dietary Fiber	1 g
Sugars	1 g
Protein	2 g

1 pound asparagus spears, trimmed, rinsed and patted dry

2 teaspoons sesame seeds

1. Preheat oven to 400°F.

2. Coat a nonstick baking sheet with cooking spray, arrange asparagus on baking sheet, and liberally coat asparagus with cooking spray and sprinkle with sesame seeds. Season lightly with salt, if desired.

3. Bake 10 minutes until asparagus is just tender.

BLACK BEANS, GRAPE TOMATOES, AND LIME

Serves: 4 • Serving Size: 1/2 cup

1	cup chopped onions
1	15-ounce can black beans, rinsed and drained
1/2	cup grape tomatoes, quartered
1	tablespoon lime juice
1/2 to 1	teaspoon ground cumin
1	tablespoon extra virgin olive oil
2	tablespoons chopped cilantro

1. Place a large nonstick skillet over medium-high heat until hot. Coat skillet with cooking spray, add the onions, and coat with cooking spray. Cook onions 4 minutes or until beginning to brown, stirring frequently. Stir in the beans, tomatoes, lime juice, and cumin. Cook 1 minute or until heated through, stirring frequently. Remove from heat.

2. Season lightly with salt and pepper, if desired. Drizzle the oil evenly over all, and sprinkle evenly with the cilantro. Do not stir. Cover and let stand 5 minutes to absorb flavors.

Exchanges/Choices

1 Starch
1 Vegetable
1/2 Fat

Calories	130
Calories from Fat	35
Total Fat	4.0 g
Saturated Fat	0.6 g
Trans Fat	0.0 g
Cholesterol	0 mg
Sodium	80 mg
Total Carbohydrate	19 g
Dietary Fiber	6 g
Sugars	4 g
Protein	6 g

DILLED WHOLE GREEN BEANS

Serves: 4 • Serving Size: 1/4 recipe

Exchanges/Choices

2 Vegetable

Calories	50
Calories from Fat	15
Total Fat	1.5 g
Saturated Fat	0.4 g
Trans Fat	0.0 g
Cholesterol	0 mg
Sodium	80 mg
Total Carbohydrate	8 g
Dietary Fiber	3 g
Sugars	2 g
Protein	2 g

1 pound whole green beans, trimmed
1 tablespoon reduced-fat margarine
2 teaspoons Dijon mustard
1/2 teaspoon dried dill weed

1. Place 2 cups water in a large saucepan, place a collapsible steamer basket on bottom of pan, arrange beans evenly on basket, and cover tightly. Bring water to a boil and steam beans 6 minutes or until just tender-crisp.

2. In a small bowl, combine remaining ingredients.

3. Place cooked beans in a serving bowl and toss with the margarine mixture. Salt to taste, if desired. Serve immediately.

BROCCOLI WITH SPICY CHEESE SAUCE

Serves: 4 • Serving Size: 1 cup

4 cups broccoli florets
4 slices reduced-fat American cheese
2 teaspoons fat-free milk
1/2 teaspoon Worcestershire sauce
1/8 to 1/4 teaspoon cayenne pepper

1. Place 2 cups water in a large saucepan, place a collapsible steamer basket on bottom of pan, arrange florets evenly on basket, and cover tightly. Bring water to a boil and steam broccoli 5 to 6 minutes or until just tender-crisp.

2. When broccoli has cooked, place cheese slices in a microwaveable bowl, cover with plastic wrap, and microwave on HIGH setting 45 seconds or until cheese has melted. Stir in remaining ingredients.

3. Arrange broccoli on a serving platter, drizzle sauce over broccoli, serve immediately.

Exchanges/Choices

1 Vegetable
1 Lean Meat

Calories	70
Calories from Fat	25
Total Fat	3.0 g
Saturated Fat	1.5 g
Trans Fat	0.0 g
Cholesterol	10 mg
Sodium	315 mg
Total Carbohydrate	6 g
Dietary Fiber	2 g
Sugars	4 g
Protein	6 g

SWEET MUSTARD-GLAZED BABY CARROTS

Serves: 4 • Serving Size: 1/2 cup

Exchanges/Choices

1/2 Carbohydrate
1 Vegetable
1/2 Fat

Calories	80
Calories from Fat	20
Total Fat	2.5 g
Saturated Fat	0.2 g
Trans Fat	0.0 g
Cholesterol	0 mg
Sodium	95 mg
Total Carbohydrate	14 g
Dietary Fiber	2 g
Sugars	10 g
Protein	1 g

1/2 cup water
10 ounces (about 2 cups) baby carrots
2 tablespoons packed dark brown sugar
2 teaspoons canola oil
1 tablespoon prepared mustard
1 to 2 teaspoons grated orange zest

1. Bring water to boil in a large nonstick skillet over medium-high heat. Add the carrots, cover tightly, and cook 7 minutes or until the carrots are tender-crisp and the liquid has evaporated.

2. Meanwhile, combine the remaining ingredients in a small bowl. Stir in the sugar mixture to the carrots. Cook 3 minutes, uncovered, until glazed, using two utensils to stir as you would a stir fry.

BAYOU SKILLET CORN

Serves: 4 • Serving Size: 1/2 cup

1 10-ounce package (about 2 cups) frozen corn kernels, thawed and patted dry

1/4 cup finely chopped red or green bell pepper

1/4 teaspoon chili powder

2 tablespoons reduced-fat margarine

1 tablespoon chopped parsley

1/2 teaspoon Louisiana hot sauce

1. Place a large nonstick skillet over medium-high heat until hot. Coat with cooking spray, add the corn, bell pepper, and chili powder and cook 3 minutes or until heated thoroughly. Remove from heat, add the remaining ingredients, and stir until well coated. Season lightly with salt and pepper, if desired.

2. Serve immediately for peak flavors.

Exchanges/Choices

1 Starch

Calories	85
Calories from Fat	25
Total Fat	3.0 g
Saturated Fat	0.8 g
Trans Fat	0.0 g
Cholesterol	0 mg
Sodium	50 mg
Total Carbohydrate	14 g
Dietary Fiber	2 g
Sugars	3 g
Protein	2 g

SPINACH AND BACON

Serves: 4 • Serving Size: 1/4 recipe

Exchanges/Choices

1 Vegetable

1/2 Fat

Calories	50	
Calories from Fat	30	
Total Fat	3.5	g
Saturated Fat	1.3	g
Trans Fat	N/A	
Cholesterol	5	mg
Sodium	125	mg
Total Carbohydrate	2	g
Dietary Fiber	1	g
Sugars	0	g
Protein	3	g

2 bacon slices, cut in very small pieces

1 9-ounce package fresh spinach leaves

2 tablespoons water

1. Place a large nonstick skillet over medium-high heat. Add bacon and cook until crisp. Remove bacon and blot on paper towels. Discard all but 2 teaspoons of the bacon grease.

2. Add spinach, water, and salt to taste to the 2 teaspoons bacon grease. Toss constantly until limp and tender, about 1 minute, using two utensils.

3. Remove from heat, crumble bacon on top, and serve.

SAUTEED ROSEMARY SPRING GREENS

Serves: 4 • Serving Size: about 1/3 cup

1 tablespoon extra virgin olive oil

4 medium garlic cloves, peeled

2 5-ounce packages spring greens, or 10 ounces baby spinach leaves

1/4 to 1/2 teaspoon chopped fresh rosemary

1. Place a large nonstick skillet over medium-high heat until hot. Add the oil and garlic and cook 2 minutes or until lightly golden. Add half of the spring greens and cook 1 minute, stirring with two utensils, as you would a stir fry.

2. Add remaining spring greens and rosemary, and 1/4 teaspoon salt, if desired, and cook 30 seconds or until just beginning to wilt.

3. Remove from heat and let stand 2 minutes to absorb flavors. Remove garlic before serving.

Exchanges/Choices

1 Vegetable
1/2 Fat

Calories	45
Calories from Fat	30
Total Fat	3.5 g
Saturated Fat	0.5 g
Trans Fat	0.0 g
Cholesterol	0 mg
Sodium	20 mg
Total Carbohydrate	3 g
Dietary Fiber	1 g
Sugars	1 g
Protein	1 g

Cook's Note

It's important to allow the greens to stand 2 to 3 minutes to allow flavors to absorb.

BROILED BLUE CHEESE ROMAS

Serves: 4 • Serving Size: 1/4 recipe

Exchanges/Choices

1 Vegetable
1/2 Fat

Calories	40	
Calories from Fat	20	
Total Fat	2.0	g
Saturated Fat	1.4	g
Trans Fat	0.1	g
Cholesterol	5	mg
Sodium	190	mg
Total Carbohydrate	3	g
Dietary Fiber	1	g
Sugars	2	g
Protein	2	g

4 Roma or plum tomatoes, halved lengthwise
2 tablespoons fat-free Italian salad dressing
1/2 teaspoon dried basil leaves
1/4 cup blue cheese, crumbled

1. Preheat broiler.

2. Arrange tomatoes on a nonstick baking sheet, cut-side up. Drizzle dressing evenly over tomatoes and then sprinkle with basil.

3. Broil 2 to 3 inches away from heat source for 1 minute. Remove tomatoes from broiler and top with cheese and salt and pepper to taste.

4. Return to broiler, turn off heat, and let stand in oven 3 minutes or until cheese just begins to turn lightly golden.

FREE VEGGIE STIR-FRY

Serves: 4 • Serving Size: 1/4 recipe

1	medium yellow squash, trimmed and cut into eighths lengthwise
1/2	medium green bell pepper, cut into thin strips
1	medium yellow onion, cut into 1/2-inch wedges, layers separated

1. Place a large nonstick skillet over medium-high heat. Coat skillet with nonstick cooking spray. Add vegetables and cook 3 to 4 minutes or until tender crisp, stirring constantly.

2. Add salt to taste. Remove from heat and let stand 1 minute before serving.

Exchanges/Choices
1 Vegetable

Calories	20
Calories from Fat	0
Total Fat	0.0 g
Saturated Fat	0.0 g
Trans Fat	0.0 g
Cholesterol	0 mg
Sodium	0 mg
Total Carbohydrate	5 g
Dietary Fiber	1 g
Sugars	3 g
Protein	1 g

CHILI-SAUTEED VEGGIES

Serves: 4 • Serving Size: about 2/3 cup

Exchanges/Choices

1/2 Starch

1 Vegetable

Calories	55
Calories from Fat	15
Total Fat	1.5 g
Saturated Fat	0.5 g
Trans Fat	0.0 g
Cholesterol	0 mg
Sodium	30 mg
Total Carbohydrate	10 g
Dietary Fiber	2 g
Sugars	3 g
Protein	2 g

1 cup pre-sliced multi-colored peppers and onions, or 1/2 cup sliced red bell pepper and 1/2 cup thinly sliced onion

1 medium zucchini, quartered lengthwise and cut into 2-inch pieces

1 cup frozen corn kernels, thawed

1 tablespoon reduced-fat margarine

1/2 teaspoon chili powder

1. Place a large nonstick skillet over medium-high heat until hot. Coat skillet with cooking spray, add the peppers, onions, and zucchini, coat the vegetables with cooking spray, and cook 6 minutes or until zucchini is tender-crisp, stirring frequently.

2. Add the remaining ingredients and cook 1 minute, stirring constantly. Season with 1/4 teaspoon salt and 1/8 teaspoon black pepper, if desired.

SNOW PEAS AND RED PEPPER SKILLET TOSS

Serves: 4 • Serving Size: 1/2 cup

1 cup chopped onion
1 cup chopped red bell pepper
1 cup fresh or frozen snow peas
1 medium garlic clove, minced

1. Place a large nonstick skillet over medium-high heat until hot. Coat skillet with cooking spray, add the onions, and cook 2 minutes, stirring frequently, using two utensils as you would for a stir fry. Add peppers and cook 2 to 3 minutes or until onions are translucent. Add the peas and season lightly with salt and pepper, if desired. Cook 1 to 2 minutes to heat thoroughly. Add the garlic, cook 15 seconds, stirring constantly.

Exchanges/Choices
2 Vegetable

Calories	45
Calories from Fat	0
Total Fat	0.0 g
Saturated Fat	0.1 g
Trans Fat	0.0 g
Cholesterol	0 mg
Sodium	0 mg
Total Carbohydrate	9 g
Dietary Fiber	3 g
Sugars	5 g
Protein	2 g

THYME-SCENTED SQUASH WITH CHEDDAR

Serves: 4 • Serving Size: 1/2 cup

Exchanges/Choices

1 Vegetable
1/2 Fat

Calories	55	
Calories from Fat	15	
Total Fat	1.5	g
Saturated Fat	0.9	g
Trans Fat	0.0	g
Cholesterol	5	mg
Sodium	65	mg
Total Carbohydrate	8	g
Dietary Fiber	2	g
Sugars	4	g
Protein	3	g

1 cup chopped onion
2 medium yellow squash, sliced
1 medium jalapeno, seeded, finely chopped, or 1/8 teaspoon dried red pepper flakes
1/2 teaspoon dried thyme leaves
1/4 cup shredded reduced-fat sharp cheddar cheese

1. Place a large nonstick skillet over medium-high heat until hot. Lightly coat the skillet with cooking spray, add the onion and coat the onions with cooking spray. Cook 4 minutes or until onions are browned, stirring frequently. Stir in the squash, jalapeno, and thyme. Coat with cooking spray, reduce heat to medium, cover, and cook 4 minutes or until squash is tender and beginning to brown, stirring occasionally.

2. Remove from heat, lightly season with salt and pepper, if desired, and sprinkle with cheese.

ORANGE AND BUTTERY ACORN SQUASH

Serves: 4 • Serving Size: 1 wedge and 2 tablespoons sauce

1 medium acorn squash, about 1 1/2 pounds
1/3 cup orange juice
2 tablespoons honey
1/4 teaspoon ground nutmeg
2 tablespoons reduced-fat margarine

1. Pierce squash several times with a sharp knife, then place on paper towels in microwave oven. Microwave on HIGH setting 1 minute. Cut squash in half lengthwise and discard seeds and membrane. Cut each squash half lengthwise into 4 wedges. Pour the juice into an 11-inch by 7-inch baking dish. Place squash, cut-sides down, in pan. Cover with plastic wrap, turning back one corner to vent (do not allow plastic wrap to touch food). Microwave on HIGH setting 10 minutes or until tender.

2. Place the squash, cut-side up, on a serving platter. Add the remaining ingredients to the drippings in the pan and stir until just melted. Spoon mixture evenly over squash wedges.

Exchanges/Choices

1 Starch
1/2 Carbohydrate

Calories	120
Calories from Fat	20
Total Fat	2.5 g
Saturated Fat	0.8 g
Trans Fat	0.0 g
Cholesterol	0 mg
Sodium	45 mg
Total Carbohydrate	25 g
Dietary Fiber	4 g
Sugars	15 g
Protein	1 g

Cook's Note

Cooking the whole squash one minute makes for easier cutting.

CREAMY CHEESE GRITS

Serves: 6 • Serving Size: 1/2 cup

Exchanges/Choices

1 Starch

1/2 Fat

Calories	95
Calories from Fat	20
Total Fat	2.0 g
Saturated Fat	1.2 g
Trans Fat	0.0 g
Cholesterol	10 mg
Sodium	220 mg
Total Carbohydrate	14 g
Dietary Fiber	0 g
Sugars	2 g
Protein	4 g

2 3/4 cups water

1/2 cup quick-cooking grits

4 slices reduced-fat American cheese

1/2 cup fat-free half-and-half

1/8 teaspoon cayenne pepper

1. In a medium saucepan, bring water to boil over high heat. Stir in the grits, reduce heat, cover tightly, and simmer 5 minutes or until most of the liquid has been absorbed.

2. Remove from heat and stir in remaining ingredients. Cover and let stand 2 to 3 minutes to thicken slightly and allow flavors to blend. Sprinkle lightly with salt and pepper, if desired.

SWEET POTATOES WITH ORANGE MARMALADE

Serves: 4 • Serving Size: 1/4 recipe

2	8-ounce sweet potatoes, pierced several times
1 1/2	tablespoons reduced-fat margarine
1 1/2	tablespoons orange marmalade
1/2	teaspoon ground cinnamon

1. Place potatoes in microwave and cook on HIGH setting for 6 minutes or until tender when pierced with a fork.

2. Meanwhile, in a small mixing bowl, combine remaining ingredients and set aside.

3. When potatoes are done, split in half lengthwise, fluff potatoes with a fork, and spoon equal amounts (about 2 teaspoons each) of the marmalade mixture on top of each potato half.

Exchanges/Choices

1 1/2 Starch

Calories	120	
Calories from Fat	20	
Total Fat	2.0	g
Saturated Fat	0.6	g
Trans Fat	0.0	g
Cholesterol	0	mg
Sodium	70	mg
Total Carbohydrate	24	g
Dietary Fiber	3	g
Sugars	10	g
Protein	2	g

GREEK POTATO WEDGES

Serves: 4 • Serving Size: 1/4 recipe

Exchanges/Choices

2 Starch

1/2 Fat

Calories	175
Calories from Fat	65
Total Fat	7.0 g
Saturated Fat	0.9 g
Trans Fat	0.0 g
Cholesterol	0 mg
Sodium	55 mg
Total Carbohydrate	27 g
Dietary Fiber	3 g
Sugars	2 g
Protein	3 g

1 pound new red potatoes (about 2 ounces each), cut into 1/2-inch wedges

2 tablespoons extra virgin olive oil

1/2 teaspoon lemon pepper seasoning

1/2 teaspoon dried oregano leaves

2 tablespoons chopped fresh parsley

1. Place 2 cups water in a large saucepan, place a collapsible steamer basket on bottom of pan, arrange potato wedges evenly on basket, and cover tightly. Bring water to a boil, cover, and steam potatoes 8 minutes or until just tender.

2. Place potatoes in a serving bowl and toss gently with remaining ingredients. Cover and let stand 3 minutes to absorb flavors.

3. Sprinkle with parsley and serve.

SOUR CREAM POTATOES WITH ONIONS

Serves: 4 • Serving Size: about 3/4 cup

2	cups water
1	pound red potatoes, sliced
1	cup chopped onions
1/3	cup light sour cream
2	tablespoons grated Parmesan cheese
2	tablespoons fat-free milk
1/4	cup chopped parsley

1. Place a collapsible steamer basket into a large saucepan. Add the water, arrange the potatoes and onion in basket, and bring to a boil over high heat. Cover tightly and steam 8 to 10 minutes or until potatoes are just tender.

2. Meanwhile, in a small bowl, combine the remaining ingredients, except parsley. Place potatoes in a shallow pasta bowl or serving platter and spoon sour cream mixture evenly over the potatoes. Sprinkle with the parsley. Season lightly with salt and pepper, if desired.

Exchanges/Choices

2 Starch
1/2 Fat

Calories	180
Calories from Fat	30
Total Fat	3.5 g
Saturated Fat	2.3 g
Trans Fat	0.0 g
Cholesterol	15 mg
Sodium	60 mg
Total Carbohydrate	32 g
Dietary Fiber	3 g
Sugars	6 g
Protein	6 g

ROUGH POTATO MASH

Serves: 5 • Serving Size: 1/2 cup

Exchanges/Choices

1 1/2 Starch
1/2 Fat

Calories	145	
Calories from Fat	25	
Total Fat	3.0	g
Saturated Fat	1.5	g
Trans Fat	0.0	g
Cholesterol	5	mg
Sodium	80	mg
Total Carbohydrate	25	g
Dietary Fiber	2	g
Sugars	5	g
Protein	5	g

1	pound unpeeled baking potatoes, diced
1/2	cup evaporated fat-free milk
2	tablespoons reduced-fat margarine
1/4	cup light sour cream
1/8	teaspoon garlic powder

1. Place 2 cups water in a large saucepan, place a collapsible steamer basket on bottom of pan, arrange potatoes evenly on basket, and cover tightly. Bring water to a boil and steam potatoes 8 minutes or until just tender.

2. Place potatoes in a serving bowl and, using whisk, mash potatoes. Add remaining ingredients and whisk until well blended. The texture will be a bit lumpy.

PASTA WITH BASIL AND PARMESAN

Serves: 4 • Serving Size: 1/2 cup

4 ounces uncooked whole-grain pasta, any shape
1 tablespoon lemon juice
1 tablespoon parsley, finely chopped
2 teaspoons extra virgin olive oil
1 teaspoon dried basil leaves
2 tablespoons grated Parmesan cheese

1. Cook pasta according to package directions, omitting any salt or fats.

2. Meanwhile, in a small bowl, combine remaining ingredients except Parmesan.

3. Place pasta in serving bowl and toss with lemon mixture. Sprinkle with Parmesan and salt to taste. Serve immediately.

Exchanges/Choices

1 1/2 Starch
1/2 Fat

Calories	140
Calories from Fat	30
Total Fat	3.5 g
Saturated Fat	0.9 g
Trans Fat	0.0 g
Cholesterol	5 mg
Sodium	30 mg
Total Carbohydrate	23 g
Dietary Fiber	3 g
Sugars	1 g
Protein	5 g

FRESH OREGANO MUSHROOM PASTA

Serves: 4 • Serving Size: 1/2 cup

Exchanges/Choices

1/2 Starch

1 Vegetable

1 Fat

Calories	100
Calories from Fat	35
Total Fat	4.0 g
Saturated Fat	0.5 g
Trans Fat	0.0 g
Cholesterol	0 mg
Sodium	10 mg
Total Carbohydrate	14 g
Dietary Fiber	3 g
Sugars	2 g
Protein	4 g

2	ounces uncooked whole-grain penne or rotini
1	tablespoon extra virgin olive oil
8	ounces sliced mushrooms
1	medium garlic clove, minced
1/2	cup finely chopped green onions
1	tablespoon oregano leaves, chopped

1. Cook pasta according to package directions, omitting any salt or fats.

2. Meanwhile, place a large nonstick skillet over medium-high heat until hot. Add 1 teaspoon of the oil, tilt the skillet to coat lightly, add the mushrooms, coat mushrooms with cooking spray, and cook 6 to 7 minutes or until lightly brown on edges, stirring frequently. Add the garlic and cook 15 seconds, stirring constantly.

3. Remove from heat and stir in the drained pasta and remaining ingredients. Toss until well blended.

TOASTED PECAN AND BROWN ONION RICE

Serves: 4 • Serving Size: 1/2 cup

1 1/4	cups water
1/2	cup quick-cooking brown rice
1	cup chopped onion
1/4	cup pecan pieces
1/2	teaspoon sugar
1/2	teaspoon ground cumin
1/8	teaspoon ground nutmeg

1. In a small saucepan, bring water to boil over high heat, add the rice, cover, and simmer 10 to 12 minutes or until water is absorbed.

2. Meanwhile, place a large nonstick skillet over medium-high heat until hot. Add the pecans and cook 2 minutes or until beginning to lightly brown, stirring frequently. Remove from skillet and set aside on separate plate.

3. Coat the skillet with cooking spray, add the onions, coat the onions with cooking spray, and cook 6 minutes or until richly browned, stirring frequently. Remove from heat, stir in the rice, cumin, and pecans and toss to blend. Season lightly with salt and pepper, if desired.

Exchanges/Choices

1 Starch
1 Vegetable
1 Fat

Calories	155
Calories from Fat	55
Total Fat	6.0 g
Saturated Fat	0.6 g
Trans Fat	0.0 g
Cholesterol	0 mg
Sodium	15 mg
Total Carbohydrate	23 g
Dietary Fiber	2 g
Sugars	3 g
Protein	3 g

DESSERTS

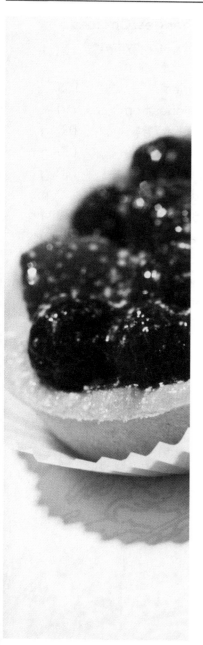

ANGEL CAKE WITH RASPBERRY CREAM AND NECTARINES

Serves: 4 • Serving Size: 1/4 recipe

3/4 cup fat-free whipped topping

3 tablespoons seedless raspberry 100% fruit spread

1/4 teaspoon almond extract

4 ounces (about 1/4 of a standard cake) angel food cake, cut in 4 slices

2 cups sliced nectarines or peaches

1. In a small mixing bowl, mix together whipped topping with fruit spread and extract.

2. Spoon equal amount (about 2 tablespoons) over each slice of cake and top with 1/2 cup nectarine slices per serving.

Exchanges/Choices
2 1/2 Carbohydrate

Calories	155
Calories from Fat	0
Total Fat	0.0 g
Saturated Fat	0.0 g
Trans Fat	0.0 g
Cholesterol	0 mg
Sodium	150 mg
Total Carbohydrate	36 g
Dietary Fiber	1 g
Sugars	21 g
Protein	2 g

BUTTERSCOTCH CHIP CAKE MIX COOKIES

Serves: 48 • Serving Size: 1 cookie

Exchanges/Choices

1 Carbohydrate
1/2 Fat

Calories	80
Calories from Fat	20
Total Fat	2.5 g
Saturated Fat	1.6 g
Trans Fat	0.0 g
Cholesterol	5 mg
Sodium	105 mg
Total Carbohydrate	13 g
Dietary Fiber	0 g
Sugars	8 g
Protein	1 g

1   18.25-ounce box spice cake mix
2   tablespoons margarine, softened
2   tablespoons water
1   large egg
2   egg whites
1   cup quick-cooking oats
1   cup butterscotch chips or raisins

1. Preheat oven to 350°F.

2. In a large mixing bowl, combine cake mix, margarine, water, egg, and egg whites. Using an electric mixer, beat on medium speed until blended. Add the oats and beat until well blended. Stir in the chips.

3. Drop by rounded tablespoons 2 inches apart onto baking sheet coated with cooking spray. Bake 8 minutes or until a few air bubbles begin to appear on top of the cookies. The cookies will not appear to be done, but they will continue cooking as they cool. Carefully remove cookies with a flat spatula and cool completely on a wire rack.

Cook's Note

You can make a smaller amount of cookies and freeze the remaining cookie dough in an airtight container for 1 to 2 weeks. Or you can bake all of the cookie dough and freeze cookies in freezer bags up to 1 month.

RUSTIC APPLE CRISP

Serves: 8 • Serving Size: 1/8 recipe

1/2 cup pecan chips (smaller than pieces)

1 pound (about 5 cups sliced) Granny Smith apples, halved, cored, and cut into 1/2-inch wedges

2 tablespoons water

1/2 teaspoon ground cinnamon

1/4 cup fat-free caramel ice cream topping

2 cups low-fat granola cereal

1. Place a large nonstick skillet over medium-high heat. Add pecans and cook 2 minutes or until just beginning to turn golden and fragrant, stirring frequently. Remove from skillet and set aside on a separate plate.

2. Cut apples in half, core, and cut in 1/2-inch wedges. Return skillet to heat. Add apples and water and cook, uncovered, 4 minutes or until just tender-crisp, stirring frequently.

3. Remove skillet from heat and sprinkle cinnamon over apples. Drizzle 1 tablespoon caramel topping over apples and stir gently. Top with granola, cover, and let stand 1 minute to absorb flavors.

4. Place remaining caramel topping in a microwave bowl and microwave on HIGH setting for 15 seconds. Drizzle over granola and top with nuts to serve.

Exchanges/Choices

2 Carbohydrate

1 Fat

Calories	195	
Calories from Fat	65	
Total Fat	7.0	g
Saturated Fat	0.8	g
Trans Fat	0.0	g
Cholesterol	0	mg
Sodium	80	mg
Total Carbohydrate	34	g
Dietary Fiber	4	g
Sugars	17	g
Protein	3	g

INDIVIDUAL STRAWBERRIES AND CREAM FRUIT TARTS

Serves: 4 • Serving Size: 3 shells

Exchanges/Choices

1 1/2 Carbohydrate
1 Fat

Calories	140
Calories from Fat	45
Total Fat	5.0 g
Saturated Fat	1.2 g
Trans Fat	0.0 g
Cholesterol	5 mg
Sodium	60 mg
Total Carbohydrate	25 g
Dietary Fiber	1 g
Sugars	13 g
Protein	0 g

1/4 cup lemon curd or apricot 100% fruit spread
12 phyllo mini shells
1/2 cup sugar-free whipped topping
1 cup quartered strawberries

1. Place the lemon curd or fruit spread in a small microwave-safe bowl, microwave on HIGH setting 20 seconds or until slightly melted.

2. Spoon 1 teaspoon of the lemon curd into each of the shells. Top with 2 teaspoons whipped topping and equal amounts strawberries in each shell.

KIWI-BLUEBERRY TARTS WITH CREAMY APRICOT GINGER

Serves: 4 • Serving Size: 1 tart

1/3 cup apricot 100% fruit spread

1 teaspoon grated ginger

2 6-ounce containers nonfat lemon yogurt with mainly low-calorie sweetener

2 ripe kiwi, peeled and diced

1 cup blueberries

1. Place the fruit spread in a small microwave-safe bowl and heat on HIGH setting 20 seconds or until slightly melted. Stir in the ginger.

2. Spoon equal amounts (about 1 1/2 tablespoons) of the fruit spread mixture into each of four ramekins. Spoon equal amounts of the yogurt over the fruit spread and top with the kiwi and berries.

Exchanges/Choices

1/2 Fat-Free Milk
1 1/2 Carbohydrate

Calories	135
Calories from Fat	0
Total Fat	0.0 g
Saturated Fat	0.1 g
Trans Fat	0.0 g
Cholesterol	0 mg
Sodium	45 mg
Total Carbohydrate	32 g
Dietary Fiber	2 g
Sugars	23 g
Protein	3 g

SWEET AND TART CHERRY PIES

Serves: 6 • Serving Size: 1 tart shell, 1/4 cup cherry mixture, and 2 tablespoons ice cream

Exchanges/Choices

1/2 Fruit
1 1/2 Carbohydrate
1 Fat

Calories	160
Calories from Fat	50
Total Fat	6 g
Saturated Fat	1 g
Trans Fat	0.0 g
Cholesterol	0 mg
Sodium	130 mg
Total Carbohydrate	28 g
Dietary Fiber	1 g
Sugars	20 g
Protein	1 g

1 14.5-ounce can tart cherries in water, undrained
3 tablespoons sugar
1 tablespoon cornstarch
1/2 teaspoon vanilla extract
1/4 teaspoon almond extract
6 mini graham cracker shells
3/4 cup fat-free artificially sweetened vanilla ice cream, or nonfat frozen yogurt (optional)

1. Combine the cherries and liquid, sugar, and cornstarch in a medium saucepan. Stir gently until cornstarch is dissolved. Bring to a boil over medium-high heat and continue boiling 1 full minute or until thickened, stirring occasionally, gently. Remove from heat, stir in the extracts.

2. Spoon equal amounts into each of the pie shells. Let stand 5 minutes to absorb flavors. Top each with 2 tablespoons ice cream and serve immediately. Serve with spoons for easy handling.

Cook's Note

Do not fill shells until it's time to serve them. Store any leftover filling covered in the refrigerator.

NO BAKE PUMPKIN CREAM

Serves: 4 • Serving Size: 1 filled ramekin

3/4 cup solid canned pumpkin

3 tablespoons sugar

1 teaspoon ground cinnamon

1/2 teaspoon ground nutmeg

1/4 teaspoon ground allspice

1 teaspoon vanilla

1 3/4 cups fat-free whipped topping

1. Whisk together the pumpkin, sugar, cinnamon, nutmeg, allspice, and vanilla in a medium bowl. Whisk in 1 1/2 cups of the whipped topping.

2. Spoon equal amounts in each of four ramekins. Top each with 1 1/2 teaspoon whipped topping.

Exchanges/Choices

1 1/2 Carbohydrate

Calories	110
Calories from Fat	0
Total Fat	0.0 g
Saturated Fat	0.1 g
Trans Fat	0.0 g
Cholesterol	0 mg
Sodium	20 mg
Total Carbohydrate	24 g
Dietary Fiber	2 g
Sugars	15 g
Protein	1 g

SWEET PUMPKIN WHIP

Serves: 6 • Serving Size: 1/2 cup

Exchanges/Choices

1 Carbohydrate

Calories	80	
Calories from Fat	20	
Total Fat	2.0	g
Saturated Fat	1.8	g
Trans Fat	0.0	g
Cholesterol	0	mg
Sodium	230	mg
Total Carbohydrate	14	g
Dietary Fiber	1	g
Sugars	3	g
Protein	2	g

1 3.4-ounce package instant sugar-free, fat-free cheesecake-flavor pudding

1 cup fat-free milk

1/2 15-ounce can solid canned pumpkin

1 teaspoon ground cinnamon

1/4 teaspoon ground nutmeg

1/2 8-ounce container sugar-free whipped topping

1. Combine the pudding and milk in a medium bowl, whisk until well blended. Stir in the pumpkin, cinnamon, and nutmeg. Gently stir in the whipped topping until just blended.

2. Serve immediately or cover with plastic wrap and refrigerate up to 48 hours.

BLUEBERRY LEMON MOUSSE WITH CRUMB TOPPING

Serves: 6 • Serving Size: 1/2 cup with 2 tablespoons berries

1 0.3-ounce package sugar-free lemon gelatin
3/4 cup boiling water
1/2 cup ice cubes
1 tablespoon lemon juice
1 cup sugar-free whipped topping
1 6-ounce container low-fat vanilla yogurt with mainly low-calorie sweetener
16 reduced-fat vanilla wafers, crushed in baggie
1 teaspoon grated lemon zest
1 1/4 cups fresh blueberries

1. Combine the gelatin and boiling water in a medium bowl and stir until completely dissolved. Add the ice cubes and lemon juice and stir until ice cubes have melted.

2. Whisk in the whipped topping and yogurt until well blended and spoon into six 6-ounce ramekins or custard cups. Toss the crushed cookies together with the lemon rind and sprinkle evenly over yogurt mixture. Spoon equal amounts of the blueberries on top.

Exchanges/Choices

1 1/2 Carbohydrate
1/2 Fat

Calories	120	
Calories from Fat	20	
Total Fat	2.5	g
Saturated Fat	1.7	g
Trans Fat	0.0	g
Cholesterol	0	mg
Sodium	105	mg
Total Carbohydrate	22	g
Dietary Fiber	1	g
Sugars	12	g
Protein	3	g

EASY SUMMER STRAWBERRIES

Serves: 6 • Serving Size: 1/6 recipe

Exchanges/Choices

1 Fruit

Calories	60
Calories from Fat	0
Total Fat	0.0 g
Saturated Fat	0.0 g
Trans Fat	0.0 g
Cholesterol	0 mg
Sodium	0 mg
Total Carbohydrate	14 g
Dietary Fiber	2 g
Sugars	11 g
Protein	1 g

4 cups strawberries
1/4 cup frozen purple grape juice concentrate
1/2 teaspoon almond extract

1. In a medium mixing bowl, combine all ingredients and toss gently. Serve immediately.

FRESH BERRIES WITH LEMON CREAM SAUCE

Serves: 4 • Serving Size: 1/2 cup berries plus 1/4 cup sauce

2 cups quartered strawberries

1/2 cup blueberries

2 teaspoons pourable sugar substitute

1 cup fat-free artificially sweetened vanilla ice cream, or nonfat frozen vanilla yogurt

2 to 3 teaspoons grated lemon zest

2 tablespoons lemon juice

1. Combine the strawberries, blueberries, and sugar substitute in a medium bowl and toss gently.

2. Place the ice cream in a microwave-safe bowl and microwave on HIGH setting 1 minute or until melted. Remove and whisk in the lemon zest and juice.

3. To serve, spoon equal amounts of the berry mixture in each of four dessert bowls. Spoon equal amounts of the sauce over each.

Exchanges/Choices
1 Carbohydrate

Calories	85
Calories from Fat	0
Total Fat	0.0 g
Saturated Fat	0.0 g
Trans Fat	0.0 g
Cholesterol	0 mg
Sodium	30 mg
Total Carbohydrate	20 g
Dietary Fiber	4 g
Sugars	12 g
Protein	2 g

PEARS WITH ORANGE'D MIXED BERRY SAUCE

Serves: 4 • Serving Size: 1 pear half plus 1/4 cup berry mixture

Exchanges/Choices

1 Fruit

Calories	80
Calories from Fat	0
Total Fat	0.0 g
Saturated Fat	0.0 g
Trans Fat	0.0 g
Cholesterol	0 mg
Sodium	0 mg
Total Carbohydrate	19 g
Dietary Fiber	3 g
Sugars	12 g
Protein	1 g

2 ripe pears, peeled, halved, and cored
1 teaspoon grated orange zest
2 tablespoons orange juice
1/2 1-pound bag frozen unsweetened mixed berries, thawed (reserving any juices)
2 tablespoons pourable sugar substitute
1/2 teaspoon ground cinnamon
1 teaspoon vanilla

1. Place the pear halves cut-side down in a microwave-safe shallow pan, such as a glass pie pan. Spoon the orange juice evenly over all, cover with plastic wrap, and microwave on HIGH setting 3 to 4 minutes or until tender when pierced with a fork.

2. Meanwhile, combine the orange zest and the remaining ingredients in a bowl, toss gently, and set aside.

3. Remove the pears with a slotted spoon and place cut-side down on a rimmed serving platter. To the pan drippings, add the berry mixture, cover with plastic wrap, and microwave 30 seconds or until warmed. Spoon evenly over the pears.

HONEY-GLAZED ALMOND PEARS

Serves: 4 • Serving Size: 1 pear half

1/2 ounce (a scant 3 tablespoons) sliced almonds
2 large pears, cut in half lengthwise and cored
2 tablespoons honey
1 tablespoon reduced-fat margarine
1/2 teaspoon vanilla

1. Place a large nonstick skillet over medium-high heat until hot. Add almonds and cook 2 to 3 minutes or until lightly browned, stirring frequently. Place on separate plate and set aside.

2. Coat skillet with cooking spray, reduce heat to medium, add honey, arrange pear halves cut-side down on top of honey, and cook 6 minutes or until pears are just tender. Remove skillet from heat, place pears cut-side up on serving platter.

3. To pan drippings, stir in margarine and vanilla until well blended. Stir in almonds and spoon equal amounts over each pear half. Serve immediately or cool to room temperature to allow flavors to blend, about 30 minutes.

Exchanges/Choices

1 Fruit
1/2 Carbohydrate
1/2 Fat

Calories	135
Calories from Fat	30
Total Fat	3.5 g
Saturated Fat	0.5 g
Trans Fat	0.0 g
Cholesterol	0 mg
Sodium	25 mg
Total Carbohydrate	27 g
Dietary Fiber	4 g
Sugars	20 g
Protein	1 g

Cook's Note

For peak flavors, serve 30 minutes after topping with the almond mixture. The flavors need the 30 minutes to absorb and blend, but any longer than 30 minutes and the almonds will soften and the flavors will begin to fade.

HOT APPLES WITH CINNAMON CREAM SAUCE

Serves: 4 • Serving Size: 1 apple half, 3 tablespoons sauce, and 1 tablespoon nuts

Exchanges/Choices

1 Fruit
1/2 Carbohydrate
1 Fat

Calories	140	
Calories from Fat	55	
Total Fat	6.0	g
Saturated Fat	1.5	g
Trans Fat	0.0	g
Cholesterol	0	mg
Sodium	10	mg
Total Carbohydrate	22	g
Dietary Fiber	3	g
Sugars	14	g
Protein	1	g

2 tablespoons raisins

2 tablespoons water

1/2 teaspoon ground cinnamon

2 medium apples (such as McIntosh or Gala), halved, cored, and skin pierced with a fork in several areas

1 cup sugar-free whipped topping

1 tablespoon sugar

1 teaspoon vanilla

1/4 cup pecan pieces (preferably toasted)

1. Place the raisins and water in a microwave-safe shallow pan, such as a glass pie pan. Sprinkle the cinnamon evenly over the raisins and place the apple halves cut-side down over the raisins. Cover with plastic wrap and microwave on HIGH setting 6 minutes or until tender when pierced with a fork.

2. Place the apples in individual dessert bowls. To pan residue, whisk in the whipped topping, sugar, and the vanilla until smooth. Cover with plastic wrap and microwave 20 to 30 seconds or until just heated.

3. Stir and spoon equal amounts of the sauce over each apple half. Sprinkle evenly with the nuts.

HOT PINEAPPLE AND BANANAS WITH ICE CREAM

Serves: 4 • Serving Size: 1/2 cup banana mixture and 1/4 cup ice cream

1　8-ounce can pineapple tidbits in its own juice, drained, reserving 1/4 cup juice

2　ripe, not overripe, medium bananas, peeled, halved lengthwise, and cut into 2-inch pieces

1　tablespoon reduced-fat margarine

1　teaspoon ground cinnamon

1/2　teaspoon vanilla

1　cup no-sugar-added vanilla or low-fat butter pecan ice cream

1. Place a large nonstick skillet over medium-high heat until hot. Coat skillet with cooking spray, add the pineapple, and cook 3 minutes or until beginning to lightly brown, stirring frequently.

2. Add the bananas, margarine, and cinnamon. Cook 1 minute, stirring constantly, using two utensils as you would a stir fry.

3. Remove from heat, add the pineapple juice and vanilla, and toss gently. Cover and let stand 3 minutes to absorb flavors.

4. To serve, spoon equal amounts in each of four dessert bowls and top each with 1/4 cup ice cream.

Exchanges/Choices

1 1/2 Fruit
1/2 Carbohydrate
1/2 Fat

Calories	145
Calories from Fat	35
Total Fat	4.0 g
Saturated Fat	1.7 g
Trans Fat	0.0 g
Cholesterol	15 mg
Sodium	45 mg
Total Carbohydrate	30 g
Dietary Fiber	4 g
Sugars	17 g
Protein	2 g

ICY COLD PEACH CREAM

Serves: 8 • Serving Size: 1/2 cup

Exchanges/Choices

1 Carbohydrate
1/2 Fat

Calories	95
Calories from Fat	20
Total Fat	2.5 g
Saturated Fat	1.3 g
Trans Fat	0.0 g
Cholesterol	15 mg
Sodium	25 mg
Total Carbohydrate	20 g
Dietary Fiber	3 g
Sugars	12 g
Protein	1 g

2 cups no-sugar-added reduced-fat vanilla ice cream
1 1-pound bag frozen peaches, slightly thawed
1/4 cup raspberry 100% fruit spread
1/2 cup white grape juice

1. Place all ingredients in a food processor and process until smooth. Spoon into individual parfait glasses for a "soft serve" ice cream effect. Store leftovers in an airtight container in freezer.

Cook's Note

You may need to let this stand 15 minutes to soften slightly before serving.

PEANUTTY BANANA ICE CREAM SANDWICHES

Serves: 4 • Serving Size: 1 sandwich

4 whole graham crackers, broken in half (to make eight 2-inch crackers)

1 tablespoon plus 1 teaspoon sugar-free fudge topping

1 tablespoon plus 1 teaspoon creamy peanut butter (not reduced-fat variety)

1/2 cup fat-free artificially sweetened vanilla ice cream, or nonfat frozen yogurt

8 (about 1/2 cup) banana slices

1. Spread 1 teaspoon of the fudge topping on each of four graham cracker squares. Spread 1 teaspoon of the peanut butter on each of the four remaining graham cracker squares.

2. To assemble, spoon 2 tablespoons ice cream on each of the fudge topping squares and top with two banana slices. Place a peanut butter square (peanut butter–side down) onto the bananas and press lightly to adhere. Repeat with the remaining ingredients.

3. Serve immediately or wrap individually in foil and freeze until needed.

Exchanges/Choices

2 Carbohydrate
1/2 Fat

Calories	150
Calories from Fat	35
Total Fat	4.0 g
Saturated Fat	0.6 g
Trans Fat	0.0 g
Cholesterol	0 mg
Sodium	140 mg
Total Carbohydrate	25 g
Dietary Fiber	2 g
Sugars	13 g
Protein	3 g

FRUIT-IN-THE-BOTTOM ICE CREAM CONES

Serves: 4 • Serving Size: 1 filled cone

Exchanges/Choices
1 1/2 Carbohydrate
1/2 Fat

Calories	115
Calories from Fat	25
Total Fat	3.0 g
Saturated Fat	0.8 g
Trans Fat	0.0 g
Cholesterol	0 mg
Sodium	40 mg
Total Carbohydrate	22 g
Dietary Fiber	3 g
Sugars	11 g
Protein	3 g

4 large strawberries, stems removed, or 1/2 of a small banana, peeled and quartered lengthwise

4 ice cream cake cones

4 teaspoons mini chocolate chips

4 teaspoons pecan chips or peanuts (preferably toasted)

2 sugar-free peppermint hard candies, crushed in a baggie (optional)

1 1/3 cups fat-free artificially sweetened vanilla ice cream, or nonfat frozen yogurt

1. Place a strawberry (or quartered banana) in the center of each cone. Spoon equal amounts of the chocolate chips, nuts, and peppermint on top of each. Spoon 1/3 cup ice cream on top of each filled cone. Serve immediately.

DOUBLE DARK MOCHA CHOCOLATE SYRUP

Serves: 9 • Serving Size: 1 tablespoon, plus 1/2 cup fruit

1/4	cup fat-free milk
2	tablespoons light corn syrup
1 1/2	teaspoons instant coffee granules
3	ounces semi-sweet chocolate chips
1/2	teaspoon vanilla
4 1/2	cups fruit of choice, such as banana slices, pineapple chunks, or strawberries

1. Place a small saucepan over medium heat. Add milk, corn syrup, and coffee granules and bring just to a simmer.

2. Remove from heat and stir in remaining ingredients until smooth. Let cool completely.

3. To serve, thread fruit on bamboo skewers or place in individual dessert dishes and drizzle chocolate sauce evenly over all.

Exchanges/Choices

1 Fruit
1/2 Carbohydrate
1/2 Fat

Calories	110	
Calories from Fat	25	
Total Fat	3.0	g
Saturated Fat	1.7	g
Trans Fat	0.0	g
Cholesterol	0	mg
Sodium	10	mg
Total Carbohydrate	22	g
Dietary Fiber	2	g
Sugars	15	g
Protein	1	g

FROZEN-OR-NOT STRAWBERRY WINE SLUSH

Serves: 6 • Serving Size: about 1 cup

Exchanges/Choices

1/2 Fruit

1/4 Alcohol equivalent

Calories	65
Calories from Fat	0
Total Fat	0.0 g
Saturated Fat	0.0 g
Trans Fat	0.0 g
Cholesterol	0 mg
Sodium	10 mg
Total Carbohydrate	10 g
Dietary Fiber	2 g
Sugars	5 g
Protein	1 g

4 cups frozen unsweetened strawberries

1 12-ounce can sugar-free ginger ale

1 cup dry white wine

1. Working in two batches, combine all the ingredients in a blender, secure lid, and puree until smooth.

2. Serve immediately in wine glasses or place in plastic container and seal tightly with lid.

3. Freeze overnight.

4. Scrape with a fork to create a shaved ice effect before serving

MONTH-LONG CRANBERRY WINE ICE

Serves: 12 • Serving Size: 1/2 cup

2 cups cranberry-raspberry juice (100% juice)
1 cup merlot, or any dry red wine
1/2 cup frozen purple grape juice concentrate

1. Place all ingredients in a 1 1/2-quart plastic container with a lid, seal tightly, and freeze overnight or at least 8 hours until firm.

2. Lightly scrape with a fork to create a shaved ice effect

Exchanges/Choices

1 Fruit

Calories	65
Calories from Fat	0
Total Fat	0.0 g
Saturated Fat	0.0 g
Trans Fat	0.0 g
Cholesterol	0 mg
Sodium	10 mg
Total Carbohydrate	13 g
Dietary Fiber	0 g
Sugars	12 g
Protein	0 g
Alcohol	2 g

Cook's Note

This stores well in the freezer for at least 1 month. Because of the alcohol, the mixture will not freeze solid.

INDEX

Smoked Sausage and Cheddar-Topped
    Grits, 23
Smoked Turkey Sausage and Peppers on
    Toasted Pumpernickel 163
Thousand Island Turkey and Mixed Green
    Salad, 43
Tuscan Pasta and White Bean Salad, 50

Veggie Dippers, 76
Veggie Salad on Romaine with Ham, 98

Weeknight Mexicali Beef and Rice, 130
White Bean and Sweet Red Pepper Salsa with
    Pita Wedges, 62
White Wine and Tarragon Scallops, 136

Zesty New Day Cereal, 8

OTHER BOOKS
BY THE ADA

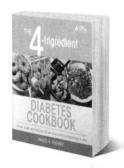

The 4-Ingredient Diabetes Cookbook
by Nancy S. Hughes
Making delicious meals doesn't have to be complicated, time-consuming, or expensive. You can create satisfying dishes using just four ingredients (or even fewer)! Make the most of your time and money. You'll be amazed at how much you can prepare with just a few simple ingredients.
Order no. 4662-01; Price $16.95

American Diabetes Association Complete Guide to Diabetes, 4th Edition
by American Diabetes Association
Have the tips and information on diabetes that you need close at hand. The world's largest collection of diabetes self-care tips, techniques, and tricks for solving diabetes-related problems is back in its fourth edition, and bigger and better than ever before.
Order no. 4809-04; New low price $19.95

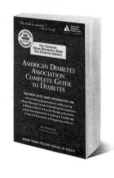

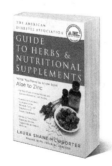

American Diabetes Association Guide to Herbs & Nutritional Supplements
by Laura Shane-McWhorter
Get reliable, unbiased information on nutritional supplements, herbs, and other natural products. This book covers 40 of the most popular alternative therapies used for diabetes, including cinnamon, garlic, ginseng, magnesium, and more! Before taking anything that may have a profound effect on your health, know what you're taking.
Order no. 4889-01; Price 16.95

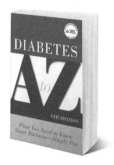

Diabetes A to Z, 6th Edition
by the American Diabetes Association

Get the ins and outs of diabetes without all of the confusing jargon. In this updated 6th edition, you'll find everything you need—from understanding A1C to getting your ZZZs, and everything in between. Own the most up-to-date recommendations by the American Diabetes Association, presented in a simple, yet informative, format.

Order no. 4801-06; Price $16.95

Holly Clegg's Trim & Terrific™ Diabetic Cooking
by Holly Clegg

Cookbook author Holly Clegg has teamed up with the American Diabetes Association to create a Trim & Terrific™ cookbook perfect for people with diabetes. With over 250 recipes, this collection is packed with meals that are quick, easy, and delicious. Forget the hassles of meal planning and rediscover the joys of great food!

Order no. 4883-01; Price $18.95

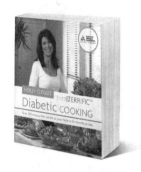

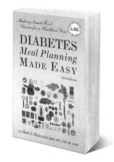

Diabetes Meal Planning Made Easy, 4th Edition
by Hope S. Warshaw, MMSc, RD, CDE, BC-ADM

This new edition of the meal-planning bestseller uncovers the secrets to healthy eating with diabetes—from the basics of what to eat to the practical skills of shopping, planning nutritious meals, and even eating healthy restaurant meals. You don't have to change your life to eat healthy, but you might be surprised to learn how eating healthy can change your life!

Order no. 4706-04; Price $16.95

To order these and other great American Diabetes Association titles, call **1-800-232-6733** or visit http://store.diabetes.org.
American Diabetes Association titles are also available in bookstores nationwide.